THE
HAPPINESS
PERSPECTIVE

THE HAPPINESS PERSPECTIVE

LEARNING TO REFRAME OUR PHYSICAL TRAUMA INTO HOPE, HAPPINESS, AND CONNECTION

FARRIS FAKHOURY
PT, DPT

NEW DEGREE PRESS

THE HAPPINESS PERSPECTIVE

Learning to Reframe Our Physical Trauma into Hope, Happiness, and Connection

ISBN   978-1-63676-109-1 *Paperback*

           978-1-63676-126-8 *Kindle Ebook*

           978-1-63676-127-5 *Ebook*

To my loving parents Amal and Nayel, my sister Mona, and brother Elias–the biggest contributors to my happiness muscle.

To all my patients. Thank you for being open, vulnerable, and allowing me to share ALL of your stories to the world. You have helped me unlock my happiness on my own personal journey in life.

~ ~ ~

CONTENTS

———

INTRODUCTION

"The greatest task for any person is to find meaning in his or her life."

VIKTOR FRANKL

Early in my career as a physical therapist, I decided to write down valuable lessons and experiences my patients have shared with me as I have treated them. Their stories and the life-changing events they go through and the drive and triumph of the human spirit never ceases to amaze me. My patients drive my passion for professional and personal growth and I am confident the lessons I learn from them can help others. I recently finished reading Bronnie Ware's book, *The Top Five Regrets of the Dying*. She initially chronicled her experiences working in palliative care on a blog platform. The top five regrets expressed to her weeks and months before the patients passed are listed below:

1. I wish I'd had the courage to live a life true to myself, not the life of others.

2. I wish I hadn't worked so hard.
3. I wish I'd had the courage to express my feelings.
4. I wish I had stayed in touch with my friends.
5. I wish I had let myself be happier.

After reading the book, I felt compelled to complement the lessons she discussed from the dying into lessons of the living. My interactions and experiences with my patients are a little different than Bronnie's. My patients have had life-changing events (stroke, brain injury, spinal cord injuries, and amputations) and now have to live with them for as long as five, ten, or even twenty years. They must learn new ways of doing things they once took for granted (as most of us do) like getting out of bed, sitting at the edge of a bed, standing, walking, feeding themselves, and so on.

Bronnie says, "Life is your own, not someone else's...it is about changing your perception and being brave enough to honor some of your own desires too."[1] This particular role has exposed me to people I never would have met otherwise. I love what I have shared with them; despite the physical and emotional challenges I must navigate. Treating the neurological patient population has made a profound impact on me. The lens through which I see my own life and the lives of those around me has shifted my perspective and my own internal dialogue of what the meaning of living truly entails. I am so thankful God has steered me onto my current path. My interactions with my patients and lessons I mention will hopefully give others the opportunity to put their energies

---

1 Bronnie Ware, *The Top Five Regrets of the Dying: A Life Transformed by the Dearly Departing* (Carlsbad: Hay House, Inc, 2011), 228.

into directions of true value to minimize the regrets of the dying Bronnie explained so beautifully.

I always knew I wanted to be in the medical field and physical therapy fit the bill. I thought it would be a job I could leave at the clinic at the end of the day. I could not have been more wrong. The connections I cultivate with my patients do not afford me the luxury of forgetting them once I leave. Most of the patients I treat are not dying, per se, but everyone is struggling with how to live with devastating and permanent injuries. I am so thankful our paths have crossed and am forever indebted to the vulnerability and trust they put in me on their individual roads of recovery.

Over the past eight years or so I have driven to work every day. I pull into the Kessler Institute for Rehabilitation campus in West Orange, New Jersey, and park my car. I grab my work bag and before I start my walk into the 152-bed hospital, I ask God to "please give me the patience and empathy to treat all my patients as I would want to be treated." I walk through the parking lot and occasionally glance into the distance to the picturesque backdrop, where the hospital sits atop a hill. I've heard stories and found it hard to believe this rehabilitation hospital once held no more than five beds in a tiny brick building back in 1948, when Dr. Henry Kessler's vision became a reality.

Dr. Kessler's story started in Newark, New Jersey, when he was born in 1896. He entered Cornell University when he was sixteen and graduated with a medical degree in 1919. He went on to get his master's and doctoral certificates from Columbia University in 1932 and 1934. Dr. Kessler volunteered to serve in the United States Navy as an orthopedic surgeon during World War II. He served as chief of orthopedics at Base Hospital No. 2 in New Hebrides, which was a rare colonial territory in which sovereignty was shared by two powers: Britain and France.

It was Kessler's vision and passion that birthed a new branch of medicine: physical medicine and rehabilitation, which included physical and emotional healing. He retired from the navy in 1946. After World War II, he became an orthopedic physician at Newark Beth Israel Hospital. His underlying goal was to educate the public in the good qualities of patients. In Kessler's book, *The Knife Is Not Enough*, he states, "this experience made me realize again the tremendous potential in the human being, potential that cannot be revealed by ordinary clinical methods."[2]

Pain, doubt, and suffering are all omnipresent when I walk through the halls of Kessler Institute. When I get into that gym and open my schedule, my colleagues and I know hope and happiness prevails and the spirit of Dr. Kessler's message is steadfast; "that rehabilitation is finally, the precious gift of hope translated into action."[3] Whether he recognized it or not at the time, Kessler's vision and purpose transcends rehabilitation medicine and being part of something bigger than myself is humbling and part of the meaning in my life.

---

2   Henry Kessler, *The Knife is Not Enough* (New York: W.W. Norton & Company, 1968), 47.

3   Ibid.

In contrast to the apparent smoothness of how Dr. Kessler's mission and vision during and post-World War II became a reality, psychiatrist Viktor Frankl's journey in finding his why and purpose was starkly different and much more turbulent; however, the underlying message has, I contend, many equal truths. Frankl was born in Vienna in 1905 and earned an MD and PhD from the University of Vienna. He began his career as a medical doctor in the late 1930s. In September 1942, he was arrested and deported. For the next four years, he spent his time in concentration camps. He has written many books, but his most infamous work is *Man's Search for Meaning*. It is based on his own experience in those camps but also the stories of the many patients he had treated. He asserts, as humans, we cannot avoid suffering but can choose how to cope with it, find meaning in it, and move forward with renewed purpose. His underlying principle is the concept of Logotherapy: our primary drive in life is the discovery and pursuit of what we personally find meaningful.[4]

I have come to realize patients respond in a myriad of different ways. It's fascinating how some patients relished the opportunity and obstacles while others retreated and played the victim. I wonder how I would react if I was recovering from a stroke, amputation, or brain injury. Would I be resilient, gritty, and battle, or would I throw in the towel and give up all hope? What is the driving force in these types of decisions? Highlighting a few insights from Dr. Frankl's journey will help set the tone for my narrative and parallel many of my experiences and stories.

---

4   Viktor E. Frankl, *Man's Search for Meaning* (Boston: Beacon Press, 1959).

Frankl's notion of finding meaning in one's life is done through three separate vehicles: in love, in work, and in courage during difficult times. While caring for others (love) and doing something meaningful (subjectively meaningful; not what others think) are realms of interest to me, my stories and insights will be more closely tied to the last of Frankl's areas of meaning through difficult times. Frankl endured some of the most unimaginable conditions in multiple concentration camps. Through it all, he was able to provide some powerful lessons—all of which are common denominators in my stories, and I hope, as you take this journey with me, will be applicable to your daily practice.

1. Everything can be taken from a man but one thing: the last of human freedoms—to choose one's attitude in any given set of circumstances.[5]
2. The sudden loss of hope and courage can have a deadly effect.[6]
3. He who has a *why* to live for can bear with almost any *how*.[7]
4. Life does not mean something vague, but something very real and concrete.[8]

I interviewed Adele Levine, the author of one of my favorite books, *Run, Don't Walk*. She said something that really resonated with me and ties into Frankl's idea of Logotherapy. "What is hard about writing about our job (being a physical

5   Frankl, *Man's Search for Meaning*, 66.
6   Frankl, *Man's Search for Meaning*, 75.
7   Frankl, *Man's Search for Meaning*, 76.
8   Frankl, *Man's Search for Meaning*, 77.

therapist treating neurological conditions and individuals who have had amputations) is that in order to do our job we have to forget our job."[9] Logotherapy regards its assignment as assisting or facilitating the patient to find meaning in his or her life. It is an awareness and not a direct result of any words, exercises, or lessons a physical therapist, psychiatrist, or friend can instill. Additionally, she said, "I don't believe in motivation; you know, I don't think you can motivate people. I think they either have it inside of them or they don't, so all I have to offer is that I can be there from nine to ten (or their scheduled physical therapy time)." Lastly, she states "we are just there to kind of help people tap into whatever is their goal."[10]

Frankl believes the role played by a Logotherapist is synonymous with an eye specialist rather than of a painter. A painter tries to convey to us a picture of the world as they see it; an ophthalmologist tries to enable us to see the world as it really is. I love this analogy. The role consists of widening and broadening the visual field of the patient so the entire spectrum of potential meaning becomes conscious and visible to him or her.[11] My Villanova soccer coach once told me it is easier to do something you want to do versus something you are told to do. I carry that in my daily mindset and try to instill it in my patients. I have learned with experience I have to read my patients and be who they want me to be.

---

9   Adele Levine, conversation with author, March 24, 2020.

10   Ibid.

11   Viktor E. Frankl, *Man's Search for Meaning* (Boston: Beacon Press, 1959), 110.

I see Logotherapy being synonymous on many levels with physical therapy.

Dr. Kessler's and Dr. Frankl's stories have helped to calibrate my perspective and the lens through which I see my own life. Experiences and the juxtaposition they both went through during and after World War II highlight the importance of finding purpose and meaning despite the circumstances with which we are presented. The stories I will be sharing with you, I believe—and pray—will guide your path in finding your meaning and purpose; a meaning and purpose already within each of us. I began to see much like Frankl saw: people who had the right perspective were able to heal themselves physically and mentally much faster. I wanted to see if these common threads were unique or part of a much larger trend. What I found changed the entire way I see healing.

While this book captures elements and stories from my own experiences as a physical therapist, I hope my stories will inspire not only professionals in the medical field but anyone going through a physical trauma to unlock a deeper meaning of purpose. My hope is this book also assists friends and family members who wish to obtain insight into the road to recovery of relatives and friends going through such traumas, potentially unlocking their own happiness along the way.

PART 1

HOW WE GOT HERE

CHAPTER 1

WHERE IT ALL BEGAN

___

The adage *we do not know where we are going without know-ing where we have been* holds true in almost every facet of our lives, and diving into the history of a profession that has influenced my life so deeply is the perfect way to start this journey. Before we rewind the clock back one hundred years, I want to share how and why I decided to become a physical therapist. I had no idea what I wanted to do with my life the day I stepped on Villanova's campus my freshman year back in 2004. Sometimes knowing what we don't want can be as illuminating as knowing what we do want. I knew I did not want to be in an office and sit in front of a computer all day. I also knew I wanted to be in the medical field in some capac-ity. I love to interact with people and hear people's stories in the process. The question became, how can I marry these together into a career?

My time at Villanova University laid the foundation for my career path. What I learned from Villanova is rooted in my experiences with the men's soccer team. The Augustinian values of unity and love call for us to care for one another and to put the needs of the community over the wants of the individual. Being part of something bigger than myself started with the soccer team and is something I still carry with me.

One of the things I remember most was in the 2008 spring soccer season. My coach told us we would be adopting an honorary twenty-seventh man to the roster: a young boy battling brain cancer. The adoption was coordinated through the Friends of Jaclyn Foundation. It is a nonprofit agency based in Chicago that helps raise awareness and funding to fight pediatric brain tumors. We spent one particular afternoon bowling with the young boy and the smile on his face is something I will never forget. In that moment, I knew I wanted to somehow be of service to others. When we make sure the lives of others are better, God will make sure ours are better too. The idea of giving back during my time at Villanova ignited a change in myself I wanted to continue fueling. I have been able to do just that through a career in physical therapy and getting the opportunity day in and day out to help others cope with life-changing injuries is something I do not take for granted.

My path to becoming a physical therapist started in 2009 and culminated with my graduation as a Doctor of Physical Therapy in 2012. I passed my licensure exam after a grueling two months of studying. After my hard work, sacrifice, and dedication in achieving my goal, I couldn't have been more excited to start my career. I accepted my position at Kessler Institute for Rehabilitation in New Jersey, an acute rehabilitation hospital, with a start date slated for the late summer heat of August 2012.

~ ~ ~

HISTORY OF PHYSICAL THERAPY

2021 is a celebration of one hundred years of the American Physical Therapy Association (APTA); an organization that has become near and dear to my heart since starting my career as a physical therapist. Below is the history of physical therapy and the evolution of the APTA:

Modern physical therapy was established toward the end of the nineteenth century in response to several factors:

- 1916: The polio epidemic became widespread in the United States, requiring the need for muscle testing and muscle re-education to restore function, growing dramatically.
- 1914-1918: During World War I, the term "Reconstruction Aide" was used to refer to individuals practicing physical therapy. The first school of physical therapy was established at Walter Reed Army Hospital in Washington DC following the outbreak of World War I.

After World War I, reconstruction aides, the predecessors to modern day physical therapists treated the countless casualties of war and getting soldiers back on their feet. As the profession continued to grow, New York University became the first to launch a full four-year science program for physical therapists. The profession continued to gain in popularity, including educational and didactic requirements.

- In the summer of 1941, six months before the bombing of Pearl Harbor, the first war emergency training course of

World War II was held at Walter Reed General Hospital. Subsequent and similar courses were started in numerous locations across the country to best treat soldiers during and after World War II.

- 1947: The association name was changed to the American Physical Therapy Association from the American Physiotherapy Association.
- 1955: The tenth anniversary of Franklin Roosevelt's death; Dr. Jonas Salk's vaccine for polio was determined to be safe and highly effective and the rest, as they say, is history.

Fast-forward ten years and Lyndon's Johnson's presidency was in full swing. The greatest impact on physical therapists was undoubtedly of the Medical and Medicaid programs. The effects of the programs were far-reaching. Millions of people previously receiving little or no health care suddenly gained access. The market was immediately in need of skilled personnel in virtually every sector of health care. Under Johnson's tenure, American ground troops were growing and the first physical therapist was part of the medical specialist corps groups.

- 1966: The first time a physical therapist and commissioned officer had been assigned deliberately to an active combat zone in Vietnam.
- 1967: Medicare and Medicaid included the services of private practitioners, including physical therapy.

Over the next few years, the profession would continue to grow and 1972 would prove to be a pivotal year for the profession:

- 1972: President Richard Nixon signed into law the Social Security Amendments, which provided independent billing authority for physical therapists. Nixon said in a statement the law was "a landmark legislation that will end many old inequities and will provide a new uniform system of well-earned benefits for older Americans, the blind and the disabled."
- 1975: President Gerald Ford signed a law that allowed and mandated education for all handicapped children. This allowed physical therapists to practice in the school system, which is a staple in the current education system to this day.
- 1990: President George W. Bush signed the Americans with Disabilities Act (ADA).

The ADA law recognized the rights of an estimated forty million Americans to equal opportunities in employment and ensured physical access to a wide range of public services and accommodations. The profession saw this as an opportunity to do important and meaningful work. The ADA calls upon the traditional skills of a physical therapist in evaluating function and pairing patients with the physical requirements of a particular activity. Simply put, employers now had someone to turn to who can better understand the modifications needed to fit certain limitations an employee might have. Again, this would serve as a springboard for the profession as whole and by the time the internet made an appearance, the APTA was ready to launch as a new frontier for the profession.

Physical therapy education has changed dramatically over the past century. Originally colleges only offered bachelor's degrees and later masters. Then, in 1996 at Creighton University, the first doctorate of physical therapy program graduated its first class of students. This change in the landscape of education for physical therapists speaks to the recognition that the complexity of patient needs requires a greater understanding of how to treat an individual in a more holistic approach.

With the turn of the century, the profession continued to set new goals to meet the ever-changing landscape of health care. In 2000, the organization and profession adopted "Vision 2020," which was a completely new path forward for the vocation. The Vision Statement for Physical Therapy 2020 states "by 2020, physical therapy will be provided by physical therapists who are doctors of physical therapy. Consumers will have direct access to physical therapists in all environments for patient and client management, prevention, and wellness services. Physical therapists will be practitioners of choice in patients' health networks and will hold all privileges of autonomous practice."[12] One of the biggest pushes and changes was evidenced-based service and care throughout the continuum of care and to improve quality of life for society.

The first ninety-nine years of the profession has surely seen its fair share of changes. This year we are witnessing another seismic shift for the profession. We are again on the front lines in a different battle. The COVID-19 pandemic has brought much to light for all of us. There is still a lot of

---

12   "100 Years: 1921-2021—100 Milestones of Physical Therapy: 2000," American Physical Therapy Association, accessed June 22, 2020.

frustration with where we are currently and where we have been the past few months. No one knows where we will eventually land but the history of the profession proves we have to look through all the uncertainty and know we are going to come out stronger.

The APTA's website says, "Where others saw limitation, we saw potential. Since our founding in 1921, we have moved forward together, with a passion and commitment to transform lives and strengthen our profession."[13] My colleagues and I have drastically shifted and changed the way we are practicing. Hand hygiene awareness has been heightened to say the least. The use of face masks is the new norm. Colleagues working in the hospital have been sent to COVID units to transfer and position patients most affected by the virus. I became a personal protective equipment coordinator for a few days in the hospital to ensure employees were safely and properly donning and doffing equipment. Many private practice clinics had to shut down for an extended period of time, including the clinic I am currently working in.

My own personal skills have shifted and grown providing care through a telehealth platform. Tele-rehabilitation is here for the long haul. We have all had a lot of time to think and reflect during this pandemic. Over the past six months, it is amazing and reassuring to think we continue to do the job set before us despite the challenges we are currently facing and have faced in the past. Physical therapy was defined during a crisis in World War I. Since then, we have consistently

13   "American Physical Therapy Association History," American Physical Therapy Association, accessed June 15, 2020.

moved forward, ensuring an exceptional patient experience along the way.

If you were to ask any colleague of mine why they chose physical therapy, I would argue the majority of them would answer in a very matter-of-fact way: to help other people. I shared and still share the same sentiment as my counterparts; however, never in a million years could I have imagined my patients would be helping me so much more than I would be helping them. The phenomenon of treating my patients using a more holistic approach has been such a profound revelation that has guided my treatment approaches. Treating the body and mind exclusively is one thing—understanding the relationship between the two is quite another.

CHAPTER 2

MIND OVER MEDICINE

——

"Much of your pain is self-chosen. It is the bitter
potion by which the physician within you heals
your sick self. Therefore trust the physician, and
drink his remedy in silence and tranquility."

KHALIL GIBRAN

The mind at its truest essence is defined as a set of cognitive faculties, including consciousness, imagination, perception, thinking, judgment, language, and memory, which is housed in the brain—the most complex of all the organs and systems in the human body. Going through my didactic work in physical therapy school, I was immediately fascinated with the power of the brain and its responsibilities of controlling the body. For an organ that weighs only about three pounds and constitutes roughly 2 percent of any human's body weight, I am constantly in awe of the capacity of the human brain. Every day I go to work, I learn something different about how the brain operates.

Early in my career, my thought process and approach was very linear as I evaluated patients. If a patient suffered a stroke and I knew what area of the brain was affected, I had an idea of how they would present to me clinically without even seeing them. I was focused on just treating the impairments of my patients versus looking at the bigger picture and considering other factors—most notably the power of the mind. I began to see patients who had the right perspective were able to unlock their happiness much faster. Trauma and the happiness perspective are centrally linked, leading to much better outcomes with my patients.

I love how Sonja Lyubomirsky defines happiness. Sonja is a professor in the Department of Psychology at the University of California, Riverside, and author of *The How of Happiness: A Scientific Approach to Getting the Life You Want*. She states "happiness has two components. The first has to do with the experience of positive emotions. The second component is that one has a sense that life is good. They are satisfied with the way one is progressing toward their life goals. Put simply: being happy in your life and being happy with your life."[14] Thoughts and perceptions affect physiology and understanding the connection between the two and reviewing the scientific research in this area is paramount in understanding this particular branch of healing.

Holistic and alternative approaches to traditional medicine have been around for centuries, but when it comes to whether these changes influence health, the question

---

14   Laurie Santos, "You Can Change," September 13, 2019, in *The Happiness Lab,* produced by Pushkin, podcast, MP3 audio, 7:30.

suddenly becomes much more intriguing. The scientific approach to the mind-body paradigm is the mind and the body are entwined. If you have a change in the body, you have a change in the mind; if you have a change in the mind, you have a change in the body. The placebo effect is defined as a phenomenon in which some people experience a benefit after the administration of an inactive substance or sham treatment. A placebo is a substance with no known medical effects, such as sterile water, saline solution, or a sugar pill.

According to Dr. Jo Marchant, an award-winning science journalist and with a PhD in genetics and medical microbiology, the placebo effect works in two ways. The first is through conscious expectation: knowledge or belief in a treatment. This is most notable and works best for symptoms you're consciously aware of, like pain, nausea, or fatigue. It includes objective visible changes like rashes and swelling. The key thing to understand is taking a placebo is not going to magically produce a chemical your body isn't normally making. A perfect example of this is insulin in a patient with diabetes.

The second is through unconscious learning processes. You take a drug several times and your body learns the physiological response to that drug. Then, if you take the placebo, your body automatically triggers that same physiological response. Drugs are one way to trigger placebo effects, but there are others, such as mindfulness or cognitive behavioral therapy. Dr. Marchant asserts when one experiences a placebo response, it's not imaginary or all in one's mind; your symptoms are eased by physiological changes just like those triggered by drugs. Through her research, she found the mind can also affect the physiological functions such as digestion, circulation, and the immune system. A prime example is the effect of stress or fear. Both can cause your heart to race or even your bowel to empty.

As I continued to explore the power of the mind on healing the body, I listened to Dr. Lissa Rankin's TEDx talk. She argues "the placebo effect is a thorn in the side of the medical field. It is an inconvenient truth that gets in the way of new and innovative treatment ideas to surface in the world of medicine."[15] Dr. Rankin is a doctor and founder of the Whole Health Medicine Institute. She has spent the last decade traveling the globe studying mind-body medicine. She highlights the spontaneous remission project, which is a database of over 3,500 case studies in the medical literature of patients who have somehow healed incurable illnesses. The case studies in this project were written up by doctors as unexplainable, which offers a peculiar peak into the mystery of medicine and the power of the mind. We have seen countless studies where the placebo effect is incredibly powerful. She set out and did research to prove the power of a healthy mind in healing the body—the premise in her book, *Mind Over Medicine*. What she found in the medical data supports the power of the mind in healing our body.

Dr. Rankin defines a healthy mind as the summation of a multitude of domains: healthy relationships, healthy creative life, financial life, healthy professional life, and healthy sex life to name a few. Attitude really matters and is evident in two studies she highlighted, indicating happy people live

15   Lissa Rankin, "Is There Scientific Proof We Can Heal Ourselves?," December 19, 2012, TED video, 0:45.

seven to ten years longer than their counterparts and optimists are 77 percent less likely to get heart disease versus pessimists. Her work explored what was happening in the brain makes the body change. At a basic level, the brain communicates with the cells in the body, using neurotransmitters released into different areas. When we are stressed, it triggers our sympathetic system, releasing chemicals like cortisol that are not supposed to be in our system for prolonged periods of time.

Conversely, when we are relaxed and in a state of tranquility, the parasympathetic system turns on and healing hormones like oxytocin, dopamine, and endorphins bathe every cell in the body. One study shows we have more than fifty stress responses in one day. The relaxation response is what researchers believe explains the placebo effect. When you get a placebo, it triggers the relaxation response. All the natural self-repair mechanisms can work their magic and come into play. The more we can tap into and activate the relaxation responses (especially after physical trauma), the more power we give our mind to nourish our body.

One particular study highlights the power of the body-mind paradigm. Researchers at Massachusetts General Hospital conducted a double-blind, randomized controlled trial of 122 patients with hypertension, aged fifty-five and older. Half were assigned to relaxation response training and the other half to a control group that received information about blood pressure control. After eight weeks, thirty-four of the people who practiced the relaxation response—a little more than half—had achieved a systolic blood pressure reduction of more than 5 mm Hg, and were therefore eligible for the next phase of the study in which they could reduce levels of blood pressure medication they were taking. During that second phase, 50 percent were able to eliminate at least one blood pressure medication—significantly more than in the control group, where only 19 percent eliminated their medication.[16]

A personal example illustrating the mind-body conundrum is through the work of Svetlana Masgutova, the originator of the Masgutova Method. This method of treatment is definitely unconventional and when I first heard of it from a colleague of mine, Mary Ellen, who uses this approach with her patients, admittedly I was extremely skeptical. Dr. Masgutova has been leading research since 1989 and has studied the influence of primary sensory-motor patterns on different aspects of development and learning. Her work focuses on the concepts of reflex integration to facilitate sensory-motor rehabilitation and emotional recovery from traumatic stress.

She gained extensive experience with post-traumatic stress disorder working with victims of the Chernobyl disaster and her work in neuro-sensorimotor reflex integration originated after a horrific train crash in Ufa, Russia, in 1989. The explosion killed 575 people and injured eight hundred more. Dr. Masgutova joined the large team of medical professionals to help the survivors. Her treatment approach is predicated on treatments using reflex patterns to reduce excitability within the nervous system and the reduction in the inflammatory

---

16   Jeffery A. Dusek et al., "Stress Management versus Lifestyle Modification on Systolic Hypertension and Medication Elimination: A Randomized Trial," *The Journal of Alternative and Complementary Medicine* 14, no. 2 (2008): 129-138.

response. The interventions she has established and shares with practitioners across the world positively impacts central nervous, immune, and endocrine systems by regulating stress hormones and neurotransmitters. At its basic form, we all have primary reflex patterns when we are born that become integrated (disappear) as we get older. When we are exposed to significant trauma, these reflexes reemerge.

My parents were in a traumatic car accident in 2017. Thankfully, they are alive and well today; however, my mom suffered the brunt of the accident, resulting in a broken hip requiring extensive surgery and months of rehabilitation. Aside from the physical traumas, my mom's underlying anxiety was exacerbated in recent years with other traumas, including her brother committing suicide a little over a year earlier, resulting in an all-time high of stress that reared its ugly head with various physical symptoms. After months of therapy, she would still have panic attacks, manifesting in episodes of shortness of breath, nausea, and intensified pressure in her neck. When traditional forms of physical therapy had reached a plateau, I decided to reach out to a Masgatova-certified clinician with the trusted help of my colleague. As a result of the trauma, the clinician unpacked how the session went and explained a few things to me; all of which highlight the impact of elevated stress (prolonged) on the body.

On assessment, she explained my mom's upper limb reflexes were very off. Her grasp, hand supporting, and hand pulling were all very off—probably a direct result of the accident and how she potentially tried to protect herself. Her therapist explained to me when she asked my mom to grab her fingers with her hands instead of her thumb coming to the front of her fist, it went to the side. This is indicative of an immature grasp pattern. Once she was going through the assessment and treatment, she also noticed my mom tended to tuck her thumb into her hand, which is a sign of stress.

This primitive reflex is present in babies but should integrate within a few weeks. If not, it is possible the baby is still under stress (from birth or more significant trauma). In adults, it is a sign of increased cortisol and stress. Her therapist proceeded to some treatment strategies for stress hormone release, performed over my mom's clothes. My mom needed a break and upon return from the bathroom, she noticed she had big red spots along her stomach and spine. Her symptoms subsided and subjectively reported her neck was feeling much better. This serves as another concrete example of how increased stress levels impact our bodies physically.

The understanding of the nervous system becomes more and more complex as scientists answer research questions and unravel new unknowns. In physical therapy school, I learned about motor imagery and the power of the mind in creating change in the body. A study by Wondrusch and Schuster-Amft illustrates just how this works. Motor imagery (MI) is defined as "a dynamic state, during which the representation of a given motor act is internally rehearsed within working memory without any overt motor output."[17] It is assumed

17   Christine Wondrusch and Corina Schuster-Amft, "A Standardized Motor Imagery Introduction Program (MIIP) for Neuro-rehabilitation: Development and Evaluation," *Frontiers in Human Neuroscience*, no. 7 (2013): 477.

action planning, action preparation, action simulation, and action observation share similar neuronal substrates. MI as a technique to improve motor performance and function has evolved in sports psychology, where a positive effect of MI training on motor performance has been shown to be highly effective. More than twenty years ago, MI as a therapeutic concept has been implemented into neuro-rehabilitation for patients with sensorimotor impairments.

The idea was to have an additional instrument besides the classical therapies to reestablish motor function. The advantage for patients has been the opportunity to train affected body parts already at an early stage of rehabilitation, when physical movement was not yet possible. As an additional advantage, patients have been able to train safely in absence of a therapist. Brain imaging and magneto-encephalography have revealed an increase in regional cerebral (brain) blood flow during motor imagery and action observation. Studies using Transmagnetic Stimulation (TMS) have reported motor imagery and action observation influence corticospinal excitability.

The framework for the mind-body paradigm is specific to recovery after trauma. The last thing I would like to bring to your attention is a concept I stumbled across during my research. Gabriele Oettingen is a professor of psychology at New York University. She is the author of *Rethinking Positive Thinking* and has numerous publications in the world of psychology. Interesting and counterintuitive to my initial thinking, she asserts the more positive thinking we do, the more likely we will not achieve the goal we are setting out to achieve. Positive fantasies are counterproductive because it makes us think we're already there. She states it is important to have times of negative thinking because the obstacles are the catalyst to help us implement and overcome what we face in life.

In her book, she discusses the notion of mental contrasting, where we ground our positive thinking and big dreams in the reality we are currently in. I love this idea for the framework of recovery. Mental contrasting IS NOT about negative thinking or constantly thinking about the obstacles you might be going through; IT IS about taking into account the obstacles YOU are facing into your plans. It is contrasting the realities of your current situation with what you want to see happen in the future. As you continue reading this book, it is important to keep this key concept at the forefront of your thinking. By doing so, it will help you determine if your vision is really achievable. If the obstacle is not possible to overcome at the moment, you can let it go and put your energy into more plausible tasks. I want to be clear this is not giving up. It is about being more efficient during the process of recovery. It helps us plan for solutions to the obstacles we are currently facing.[18]

The importance of the mind and the science behind it is out there, as I have highlighted in a variety of different avenues. Knowing what we know about the power of the mind and the impact it can have on our bodies, WE HAVE TO THINK BETTER! I have heard happiness is a choice and choosing happiness sounds pretty easy to me—but how do we choose

---

18   Laurie Santos, "Don't Accentuate the Positive," October 29, 2019, in *The Happiness Lab*, produced by Pushkin, podcast, MP3 audio, 19:45.

it, and, more importantly, sustain that choice? Happiness is more than a choice. It has to be. My experiences have taught me happiness is a perspective that entails a variety of different characteristics. The patients I have treated have taught me how to unlock this happiness perspective by turning their traumas into triumph. Throughout the process, they have helped me in my journey to unlock my own happiness, and I am confident it will help you begin to unlock yours.

CHAPTER 3: PART 1

GIVING CARE

In 2014, three friends and I went to Brazil for the FIFA World Cup. One day we took a ride with a local on a four-wheeler to explore the area of Porto de Galinhas, where we were staying. As we were traversing the narrow roads near the beach, a surfboard in front of a small house caught my attention. The surfboard read in Portuguese: "Conheci um homem tao pobre mas tao pobre que ele so tinha dinheiro." The direct translation to this is, "I met a man so poor—so poor that all he had was money." In the previous chapter, I defined happiness as a measure of how much one likes the life they are living and how much enthusiasm one feels when they wake up every day. This has nothing to do with material acquisitions or how much money someone has. Happiness is a perspective we are all in control of and the decision is ours—regardless of the hand we are dealt.

Gaining the happiness perspective is possible if you surround yourself with the right people in the right environment. In part one of this chapter, I shed light on the continuum of care after trauma as well as the importance of caregivers in the role of recovery. The reality of working with this patient population as a physical therapist inevitably leads to cultivating relationships with their caregivers to assist in recovery. I cannot stress the power and importance of a caregiver in the recovery process.

In part two of the chapter, I highlight four patient diagnoses: cerebral vascular accident (stroke), traumatic brain injury (TBI), amputations, and spinal cord injury (SCI). My goal is to provide insight into various resources to assist patients and loved ones in navigating through such vulnerable and trying times. Choosing the right key is the first step to unlock your happiness perspective. If you or someone you know is going through any one of these medical conditions, I am confident this will be the first step in recovery. Once you pick the key that fits your situation and start to implement the four main characteristics highlighted in the subsequent chapters, I am certain happiness awaits. The number one thing to under-stand as you start your road to recovery, regardless of the diagnosis, is you are not alone! I hope the following resources will allow you to shift your perspective and let healing begin.

The continuum of care and where this patient population will go during recovery varies, however. Reviewing the options is important to get some insight into these settings and what to expect. Once someone has a stroke, TBI, SCI, or amputation, they will most likely start their medical journey at an acute care hospital for a few days or weeks, depending on severity. Once medically stable and appropriate, a patient will most likely be transferred to one of three places: an acute inpatient rehabilita-tion facility (IRF), a subacute facility, or a long-term acute care hospital (LTACH). If a patient goes directly home, they may get therapy in the house or go to outpatient therapy if needed. This would be appropriate for any individual who may have minimal physical impairments and is safe enough to return home.

The table below highlights the difference between admissions to post-acute care facilities. To prevent the misuse and potential overuse of these services, there are rules in place to ensure transfers to these facilities are appropriate. Knowledge is power, so discuss your options with the case workers in the hospital and do some research yourself. I always tell my patients to try and ask at least three questions when offered an option in their health care interactions.

	SUBACUTE CARE	IRF	LTACH
Type of Care Provided	• Skilled nursing services for the short term on a daily basis in an inpatient setting	• Intensive rehab therapy in an inpatient hospital • Patient expected to benefit from 3 hours of therapy/day (5 days a week)	• Continued hospital level of care
Daily Therapy Requirements per patient	1-2 hours	> 3 hours	Variable
Average length of stay	27 days	13 days	26 days
Typical medical Conditions	• Heart Failure • Joint Replacement • Kidney and Urinary Tract infections • Septicemia	• TBI • Amputations • SCI • Stroke • Most Neurological Conditions • Multi-trauma	• Complex Wounds • Mechanical ventilation weaning • Very Complex Medical Conditions

Figure 1. Richard G. Stedanacci. "Admission Criteria for Facility-Based Post-Acute Services," *Annals of Long-Term Care: Clinical Care and Aging* 23, no. 11 (2015): 18-20.

My experiences in treating these diagnostic groups are in the outpatient setting, which is attached to an inpatient rehabilitation facility. By the time I see my patients, they are at the tail end of their recovery with regards to the continuum of care. As a general rule, in outpatient I work with my patients on a myriad of different impairments and functional limitations depending on how the patient presents to the clinic. I will work on things like gait (walking) training, strengthening, balance (both sitting and standing), range of motion, flexibility, and bed mobility.

Regardless of where you go after the acute care phase, the transition from the hospital is not an easy one. There is a lot of coordinating that needs to take place and the more you know, the more informed decisions you can make.

While this book provides ways to unlock happiness, I believe it is important to set expectations and be brutally honest during this process of rehabilitation. Some of the stories I provide might not be the easiest to hear, because the reality is—and I truly believe this—none of my patients will EVER be 100 percent back to where they were. As soon as we turn our attention to the past, we lose sight of the present; the more we strive to be like our old self, the less we are able to improve and move forward.

I interviewed Eric LeGrand who was a Rutgers University football player. He suffered a career-ending spinal cord injury in a game on October 16, 2010, leaving him paralyzed from the neck down. Since his injury, Eric launched Team LeGrand, which is a branch of The Christopher & Dana Reeve Foundation, raising money for SCI research. He has become an author, sports analyst for ESPN, and motivational speaker. He was recognized by *Sports Illustrated* with "The Best Moment of 2011." What I love most about the recipient of the Jimmy V Award for Perseverance at the ESPY Awards in 2012 is his authenticity. Every time I talk to him, I can feel what he is saying. He truly believes in his mission—to find the end zone to cure SCI. I asked him if he had any words of wisdom as I went through my journey in writing a book.

He said, "You want to be able to share stories and captivate your audience. Don't be afraid to go into the negative things that do happen because people do want to hear the negative stuff that happens. Despite the bad things that happen, there can always be a good outcome."[19] Despite how dark some of the stories I share may be, there is always light at the end of the tunnel.

A key member of the team who helps my patients start to see the light are those who care for them and are often overlooked in the value and impact they have. A caregiver can be any unpaid or paid member of a person's social network who helps them with activities of daily living after some sort of health condition, rendering an individual in need of assistance. I have come across countless caregivers who assist my patients with a plethora of activities, including transferring out of bed or a chair, bathing, arranging medical appointments, getting dressed, doing laundry, buying groceries, and the list goes on and on. I have come to notice there is a marked difference between being an aforementioned caregiver versus

---

19   Eric LeGrand, conversation with author, March 27, 2020.

actually giving care. When you are giving care, one gives for the simple fact they want to—unconditionally.

In my interview with Eric LeGrand, I asked him about his experiences with caregivers and his explanation was the perfect summation. His insights are specific to a caregiver who is not a loved one or family member. He said, "You (as a caregiver) are doing this for the patient and not the paycheck. Everyone comes from a different walk of life. Some people may have an attitude and some people may be a bitch to deal with each and every day, but try to put yourself in their shoes and see what they are going through and dealing with and always keep that level-headed mind. Eventually your patient will see that whatever they are trying to do to push you away, it is not affecting you. Then they will adapt to you and trust you and you both can be on the same page."[20]

Giving care unconditionally is not an easy task. It is a constant challenge. You will have good days and you will have bad days. My personal experience in providing care for my mom after her accident was humbling and I now have a deeper appreciation for just how powerful and important this role is. Whether you are caring for a loved one or you give care as a profession, the impact you have in helping others unlock their happiness is integral during the recovery process.

Below is a list of questions I provided to the wife of a patient of mine illustrating the power of giving care to a loved one and the impact it can have, not only on the patient, but also

---

20   Ibid.

on the individual providing the care. Her husband suffered an above-knee amputation as well as a significant brachial plexus (nerves that supply the arm) injury, essentially leaving his arm completely paralyzed on the same side he had his leg amputated.

What have you learned most about yourself?[21]

"I am stronger, braver, and more confident than I thought. My husband really did the bulk of taking care of the house, yard, cars, pool, shopping, bills, etc., and I had to assume many of those responsibilities as well as caring for his needs. I am not saying it has been easy and there have been many moments of frustration, anger, tears, and wanting to run away. I read somewhere that when you come through a storm, you do not emerge the same person and I have truly changed and have learned to rely on myself so much more than I ever did. I have learned that I need to try to be a more positive person and stop trying to control every single thing. I need to live in the moment. This is still a work in progress. I also realize that I am scared of getting sick myself, not only worried about my husband needing me, but also about who will care for me. I know that this is not living in the moment, but it is a valid concern."

What would you tell a caregiver about to start the process?

"Let yourself feel whatever you are feeling. It is natural to feel angry, scared, and question why this had to happen. Go see a therapist...find a good one. You can talk to friends and family and cry all you want, but sometimes their advice or

---

21   Patient's wife, email message to author, July 29, 2019.

encouraging words can just be annoying. I got sick of hearing it could be worse or things will get better—just look for the break in the clouds. No one truly understands if they haven't lived your journey and have seen the challenges your loved one faces every day doing the simplest task. Take as much help as is offered. Getting away for a break will refresh you and allow you to have the patience to return to your loved one. It gives you something to look forward to which is so very needed. It is so very difficult to let yourself be happy when you see how your loved one's life forever changed and your total focus in life is now on his needs."

I want to acknowledge all the caregivers out there, including family members. Thank you for all you do to help patients get through their days. The selflessness I see exhibited on a daily basis from the caregivers I interact with is truly inspiring and something that helps me recharge my batteries and makes me want to give more. I truly feel giving is contagious. Even though you are providing help to others, please do not forget to help yourselves as well so you are able to give to those you are assisting. I know how hard and tiring it can be to care for a loved one or for someone you have never met. Be gentle and kind to yourselves so your compassion will be best received by those for whom you care. When you feel like you can no longer take any more in this crazy journey as a caregiver, GIVE!

DIAGNOSTIC KEYS

"When I look at the human brain
I'm still in awe of it."

BEN CARSON

STROKE

How can a part of our body that weighs a little over three pounds be the driving force to give the capacity for thought, feelings, emotions, memories, and our overall view of the world in which we live?

This is a question I ask myself routinely and the power of the human brain is something I see on display on a daily basis. I am constantly in awe of the human mind and have been since I started my didactic work in physical therapy school and at my job. Every day I go to work, I learn something new about how the over eighty billion neurons in our brains operate. It is very oxygen hungry and requires about a quarter of the oxygen in the human body. The brain tissue is supplied with oxygen-rich blood, glucose, and other nutrients through an intricate network of arteries, and any disturbance in this system results in a cerebrovascular accident (CVA), known as a stroke.

Deficits and impairments seen after a stroke depend on three main things: LOCATION, LOCATION, LOCATION! The example I like to use is the subway system in New York City which, by the way, has twenty-one tracks and serves 1,200 trains a day. If there is a complete disruption at this train station, the effects are felt throughout Manhattan, Long Island, New Jersey, Brooklyn, Queens, Philadelphia, Boston, and even Washington DC. Let's say there is a blood clot or bleed at the "Penn Station" of the brain; the repercussions will be catastrophic. However, if there is a bleed or blockage in a tiny artery that supplies a part of the brain responsible for sensation in your arm, you can only have sensory loss in your arm with no other problems. Location is key and it is amazing to me how every stroke manifests itself in many different ways.

In December of 1995, Jean-Dominique Bauby, the forty-three-year-old editor of French *Elle*, suffered a massive stroke that left him completely and permanently paralyzed, a victim of what is known as "locked-in syndrome." Like Bauby describes in his memoir, *The Diving Bell and the Butterfly*, most people have never heard of this part of the central nervous system (which includes the brain and spinal cord), known as the brain stem.

I treat a myriad of neurological conditions, but this particular diagnosis is one of my most feared. The brain stem is the connecting structure from the brain to the spinal cord and all volitional movements in the human body. A stroke that wipes out this vital structure is indeed catastrophic. Paralyzed from head to toe, the patient, mind intact, is imprisoned inside his or her own body, unable to speak or move. *The Diving Bell and the Butterfly* is an incredible account of a man's journey after his fateful day.[22] It was written by his ability to communicate through blinking to indicate letters to form words and sentences.

Stroke

DEFINITION

A stroke happens when blood flow to the brain is blocked. This prevents the brain from getting oxygen and nutrients from the blood:
- Hemorrhagic - Bleed
- Ischemic - Blockage

Risk Factors

- Hypertension
- Smoking
- Family History
- Diabetes
- High Cholesterol
- Obesity

Fast facts

- A stroke happens every 40 seconds
- 25% of strokes occur in people under the age of 65
- 800,000 People in the United States experience a stroke every year

F.A.S.T

Can identify someone may be having stroke:
- **F** - Face
- **A** - Arms
- **S** - Speech
- **T** - Time
- Call 9-1-1

Types

Hemorrhagic 20%

Ischemic 80%

Team Members

- Neurologist
- Orthotist (Makes Brace)
- Physical Therapy
- Physiatrist
- Speech/Cognitive Therapy
- Occupational Therapy
- Psychological Services
- Wheelchair
- Adaptive Equipment

Figure 2. "Stroke," National Institute of Health, accessed April 20, 2020.

---

22   Jean-Dominique Bauby, *The Diving Bell and the Butterfly* (New York: Vintage International, 1997), 4.

CLINICAL PEARL

One particular patient, treated by a colleague of mine, suffered a stroke resulting in locked-in syndrome. I see her regularly and it is an incredible and amazing refresher for me on a weekly basis of the true beauty of the human mind. Her husband is there every session to assist with communication using the aforementioned blinking system.

I remember a conversation she was having with her husband in the gym; again the conversation is had by her ability to blink and her husband forming words to produce sentences:

- 1, a, b, c, 1, 2, 3 t, u, v, 1, 2, f, g, h, with her husband so seamlessly finishing her words as she was blinking to him. I chimed in. I do not remember specifics of the conversation; however, I know I had just returned from visiting my sister in Dubai. I decided to jump in the conversation and apparently she was not happy with what I had to say. She indicated to her husband she wanted to say something so she started blinking and her husband started forming words with the letters she was indicating;
- 1, 2, g, 1, 2, 3, l, m, n, o, 1, a, b, 1, a, 1, a, b, c, 1, 2, g, h, i, j, k, 1, 2, 3, 4, t, 1, 2, 3, l, m, n, o, 1, a, b, c, d, 1, 2, 3, 4, 5, t, u: "Go back to Dubai!" her husband finally gathered after going through their code. The entire gym started laughing.

Interacting both verbally and non-verbally with people is a true joy of mine and I am in constant awe of my patients and the challenges they overcome daily. I am so blessed to do what I love, and hope others don't settle in their personal journeys. One thing that sticks with me is how she was able to keep such a positive sense of humor during her physical therapy sessions and beyond.

In *The Diving Bell and the Butterfly,* the author describes the body as the diving bell, being so heavy, and describes the mind as a beautiful and free butterfly making the diving bell less oppressive. There is so much to do, describes the author. "You can wander off in space or in time. You can visit the woman you love, you can build castles in Spain, discover Atlantis, realize your childhood dreams and adult ambitions."[23] His account, much like this patient's, speaks to the liberating power of consciousness—a privilege I hope you cherish and never take for granted.

~ ~ ~

TRAUMATIC BRAIN INJURY

The National Institute of Health defines a traumatic brain injury (TBI) as a form of acquired brain injury that occurs when a sudden trauma causes damage to the brain.[24] It can happen when the head suddenly and violently hits an object or when an object pierces the skull and enters the brain tissue. Symptoms of a TBI can be mild, moderate, or severe depending on the extent of the damage to the brain. Concussions are a type of mild TBI. A person with a mild TBI may remain conscious or may experience a loss of consciousness for a few seconds or minutes. Worst-case scenario is a severe TBI where a patient completely loses consciousness for extended period of time. Depending on the mechanism of injury and what is going on with the actual brain tissue, surgical intervention may be warranted if there is excessive pressure on the brain.

---

23   Bauby, *The Diving Bell and the Butterfly,* 5.

24   "Traumatic Brain Injury," National Institute of Health, accessed March 20, 2020.

The most common procedure I have seen is called a decompression craniectomy. This is done to allow the swelling brain room to expand. As you can see, the spectrum within this diagnosis varies greatly. The diagram below does a great job of explaining, in basic terms, this particular diagnosis.

TBI
Traumatic Brain Injury
DEFINITION

Traumatic brain injury (TBI), a form of acquired brain injury, occurs when a sudden trauma causes damage to the brain. TBI can result when the head suddenly and violently hits an object pierces the skull and enters brain tissue. A concussion is defined a type of brain injury.

Fast facts

• 1.5 Million people suffer a TBI a year

• in 2004, an average of 155 people died each day in United States from injuries associated with TBI

• 5.3 Million people living with TBI in the United states

Causes

• Falls
• Motor Vehicle Accident
• Violence
• Sport
• Recreational Activities

Symptoms

• Cognitive function including attention and memory impairments
• Loss of consciousness
• Motor function deficits including weakness, balance, coordination
• Behavior Changes
• Vision Changes
• Headache
• Lethargy
• Fatigue
• Agitation

Team Members

• Neurologist
• Orthotist (Makes Brace)
• Physical Therapy
• Physiatrist
• Occupational Therapy
• Psyhological Services
• Wheelchair
• Adaptive Equipment

Figure 3. "Traumatic Brain Injury," National Institute of Health, accessed March 20, 2020.

CLINICAL PEARL

There are a myriad of possible effects after a traumatic brain injury. I interviewed a friend who is also a coworker and physical therapist. Shannon, who is a clinical specialist in the traumatic brain injury floor of the inpatient rehabilitation facility where we work. She has nine years of experience working with this patient population. Like Eric LeGrand recommended, I wanted to be sure to share what goes on early on the rehabilitation process in the worst of cases.

When someone has a significant brain injury, they can be in a state known as severe disorder of consciousness (SDOC). At a basic level, this means a patient is at an altered state of consciousness. Shannon explained early in the rehabilitation process, evaluations are performed daily to see how much a patient can understand. There is a formal scale inpatient therapists use called the coma recovery scale (CRS Scale). They check to see if a patient can do simple commands.

I asked, "What kind of simple commands?"

She said questions like, "Can you open your eyes? Can you kick your leg out straight? Can you open your hand? Can you take the ball?"

The next thing they typically look for is a patient's ability to communicate in some way. We are looking for any sign of response, whether it is a head shake, nod, thumbs up, or thumbs down. The following examples were shared by Shannon:

"Is your name Joe?"

"Are you a boy?"

"Are you a girl?"

Aside from volitional or voluntary types of responses, if a patient is more involved and unable to perform the above mentioned tasks, we look for more reflexive reactions. What we mean by this is where a patient is given a noxious (painful) stimulus to see if they are able to reflexively pull away from the pain.

Shannon says, "We just hope that it progresses to the point where the reflexive pull away then turns in to the patient maybe reaching over to the localized pain and eventually providing some verbal response or even pushing the therapist away."[25]

I wanted to highlight this small piece early in the recovery process to shed some light on what it really looks like, how serious a brain injury can be, and what to expect early in the recovery if the injury is this significant. It is important to recognize and realize most of the patients who have suffered a brain injury usually fall in the gray area of not minimally conscious, but certainly not returned to the way they were before.

Despite the potential severity of a brain injury, recovery happens at various rates and to varying degrees. The last question I asked Shannon sheds light on the potential in recovery.

I asked, "What is the best outcome you have ever seen? SDOC patient to fully emerge?"

She highlighted a patient who was twenty years old and struck by a car. He needed a craniotomy (removal of part of skull for some time) to release the pressure on his brain. He came in as an SDOC patient. She recounted her interaction with the

---

25   Shannon Motisi, conversation with author, April 15, 2020.

patient's mom, who was crying hysterically, in one of their earliest encounters. The mom explained how most of the doctors believed her son would never be able to walk or talk again.

Shannon said, "The patient emerged at a quicker pace than normal and now he is substitute teaching, coaching basketball, and completely independently physically."[26] She described he has some cognitive difficulties, and despite the miraculous recovery physically, the family still says he is not the same person.

The most important thing to understand throughout this whole process I firmly believe in and echoed by the sentiments of Shannon is these individuals are NEVER the same as they were prior to the brain injury. She says, "The one thing I wish that families could know right away is that no matter how good the recovery is, they are probably not going to be the exact person before the injury."[27] While this insight might not be the easiest to hear, it is the key in beginning the healing process toward a new happiness.

~ ~ ~

AMPUTEE

Individuals who have had an amputation are categorized by the level at which their amputation occurred. Outcomes and functional independence vary greatly depending on this level. Patients keep their prosthesis on through a suspension system, which can have a number of different options, each with pros and cons. There is no cookie-cutter recipe for this

---

26   Ibid.

27   Ibid.

process. Before I started my career, I thought most amputations occurred as a result of war and my immediate correlation was with veterans. More light has been shed on individuals with limb loss in unfortunate and recent events such as the Boston Marathon bombing, which resulted in numerous people needing amputations to their lower extremities. The reality of amputations is traumatic amputations account for about 45 percent, while diabetes (DM) and vascular disease (PVD) account for about 54 percent with the remaining 2 percent due to congenital and cancer.[28] I have outlined what I believe to be the most important aspects in the following image.

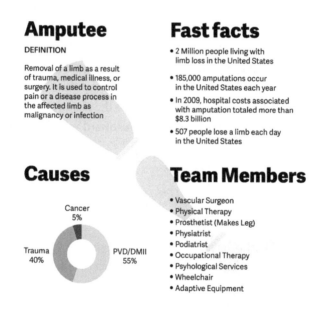

Amputee

DEFINITION

Removal of a limb as a result of trauma, medical illness, or surgery. It is used to control pain or a disease process in the affected limb as malignancy or infection

Fast facts

• 2 Million people living with limb loss in the United States

• 185,000 amputations occur in the United States each year

• In 2009, hospital costs associated with amputation totaled more than $8.3 billion

• 507 people lose a limb each day in the United States

Causes

Cancer 5%

Trauma 40%

PVD/DMII 55%

Team Members

• Vascular Surgeon
• Physical Therapy
• Prosthetist (Makes Leg)
• Physiatrist
• Podiatrist
• Occupational Therapy
• Psyhological Services
• Wheelchair
• Adaptive Equipment

Figure 4. "Limb Loss," National Institute of Health, accessed July 15, 2020.

28   "Limb Loss Statistics," The Amputee Coalition of America, accessed July 15, 2020.

CLINICAL PEARL

The most common misconception I have noticed with this patient population is patients think the prosthesis (leg) they get will do the work for them and "walk" for them. Functional outcomes and independence is much more favorable for a patient who has lost their leg below the knee versus above the knee. This is because a patient still has their own knee with a below-knee amputation. Learning to use a prosthesis when a patient lost their leg above the knee becomes more challenging as the patient now has to learn how to control a fake knee. There are many companies and vendors who sell prosthetic feet and knees and it is important to understand and look at all the options and ASK QUESTIONS! You have the right as a patient to ask questions and if you do not get along with the prosthetist (person making your leg), go to another one. You have to be comfortable with whom you work to set you up for success.

To comfortably wear a prosthesis, patients will use what is called a liner to put on their leg to protect the skin from the pressures of a hard socket the leg goes into. In a well-fitting socket, the pressure is distributed throughout the whole leg and not just one point, which helps with putting weight on that leg as the patient starts to learn to walk. Another important point to understand is even with a perfectly fitting socket, the volume or size of their leg will continue to change as they are walking and contracting muscles. It is one of the most frustrating components to understand for a patient as well as teach as a clinician. Patients will have to add socks to accommodate the change in volume for their leg. The socks patients use vary in thickness so they will have to use and change socks routinely throughout the day. If the leg is fitting poorly, it can lead to skin issues and significant setbacks during the rehab process.

Working with individuals who have lost a leg and teaching them how to use their prosthesis is a true joy of mine. Teaching my patients and their caregivers this word is always a favorite moment for me and the words I have heard my patients say are quite comical.

"I have to wear a prostitute?" My patients routinely ask me.

"Not a prostitute! A PRAS-THEE-SUS." I respond, often laughing.

The road to recovery for this patient population is multifaceted, long, and arduous for many reasons. The most obvious is the physical appearance. We live in a world where we are constantly concerned with what others think based on our physical appearance. Missing a limb brings attention to a significant physical difference that can be challenging for patients to overcome. The most interesting to me is the notion of a common symptom individuals with limb loss face: phantom pain or sensations. The human brain still thinks that part of the body is still there and continues to send signals. It is not uncommon for the patient to tell me they feel like their foot is itching even though the foot is not there.

The last clinical note worth discussing is the advances in care. I mentioned the socket and how the patient will put their leg into it. There is now a new procedure called osseointegration. This procedure implants a titanium rod into the bone of a patient. They can attach the prosthesis directly to the rod now implanted into the bone, eliminating the socket altogether. The best way to think of this procedure is similar to dental implants, where screws are put into your jawbone and, once the screw is stable and secured to the bone, the tooth implant can be used. It is the same concept behind this new procedure in the prosthetic world.

No matter what type of amputation, the new reality is a life-long process. You are in control of how you respond and begin to take your first steps and the more you know the better decisions you can make.

~ ~ ~

SPINAL CORD INJURY

Spinal cord injury (SCI) is a condition that can range in a variety of impairments depending on the severity and location. SCI usually happens to active people who, at one moment, are in control of their lives, and in the next moment, are paralyzed. Like many of the previous diagnoses described, patients need a well-coordinated, specialized rehabilitation program outlined below. SCI occurs when the spinal cord is damaged as a result of trauma, disease processes, or congenital defects. There are complete and incomplete injuries.

The spinal cord is about the size of a penny in diameter that conducts nerve signals to be sent from the brain down the spinal cord to the rest of the body. If there is a complete injury, all the tracks are damaged. If a patient suffers an incomplete injury, then a few tracks may be preserved and some signals can still be delivered along those tracks. In very basic form, the spinal cord is made up of thirty-one segments: eight cervical (neck), twelve thoracic (mid-back), five lumbar (low back), five sacral, and one coccygeal. A pair of spinal nerves leaves each segment of the spinal cord and these nerves provide signals to tell our muscles to move. The graph below sheds some light on key facts about SCI.

SCI
Spinal Cord Injury

DEFINITION

A spinal cord injury usually begins with a sudden, traumatic blow to the spine that fractures or dislocates vertebrae. The damage begins at the moment of injury when displaced bone fragments, disc material, or ligaments bruise or tear into spinal cord tissue

Fast facts

- 294,000 people living with SCI in the United States

- 78% of new cases are Male

- 1970s length of stay in rehabilitation hospital was 98 days and today only 31 days

Types

- **Complete SCI**
  spinal cord cannot send any signals past level of injury

- **Incomplete SCI**
  some signals are able to pass the level of injury

Terminology

- **Tetraplegia**
  some level of paralysis in all 4 limbs
- **Paraplegia**
  some of level of paralysis in legs only

Causes

- Falls
- Motor Vehicle Accident
- Violence
- Sport
- Recreational Activities

Team Members

- Neurologist
- Orthotist (Makes Brace)
- Physical Therapy
- Physiatrist
- Occupational Therapy
- Psyhological Services
- Wheelchair
- Adaptive Equipment

Figure 5. "Spinal Cord Injury," National Institute of Health, accessed June 14, 2020.

CLINICAL PEARL

I mentioned the spinal cord is about the size of a penny in diameter. There are clinical syndromes or distinct clinical specific signs and symptoms that can result in incomplete injuries. If the spinal cord is not completely cut, there is a likely one of the following syndromes:

1. Central cord syndrome: Where the middle of the spinal cord is compromised. Most incomplete injuries result in this syndrome.
2. Anterior spinal artery syndrome: Usually caused by flexion (forward bending of the spine) injuries.
3. Brown-Sequard syndrome: Usually a result of penetrating injuries such as gunshots or stab wounds. This results in only half of the spinal cord being damaged.
4. Posterior cord syndrome: This particular syndrome is rare and usually occurs by some sort of compression from a tumor.
5. Cauda Equina syndrome: This occurs with injuries at or below the L1 segment of the spine which results in paralysis below in the legs.[29]

There are many complications that can arise after a spinal cord injury and being aware of these potential complications can make all the difference during the rehabilitation process. The leading cause of death after SCI is pneumonia or a blood clot in the lungs, known as a pulmonary embolism.[30] I bring this up to highlight it is important to know this information to minimize them from happening. We don't know what we don't know. Knowledge is power and having this insight can help prevent complications moving forward.

---

29 Darcy Umphred, *Neurological Rehabilitation* (St. Louis: Mosby Elsevier, 2007), 607.

30 Ibid.

Another complication worth noting is autonomic dysreflexia. Being aware of this complication can literally save someone's life as it is a medical emergency. If there is a complete injury of the spinal cord, the patient loses not only the ability to move, but also the ability to feel anything below the level at which the injury occurred. Let's say you have something as innocuous as an ingrown toenail. You and I will be able to feel the pain and take care of the problem. Someone who has a spinal cord injury potentially cannot feel the pain. The ingrown toenail now becomes infected, the infection spreads into the blood, and there is a sudden rise in the patient's blood pressure. The patient begins to sweat profusely, gets a severe headache, and becomes flush in the face. Next, call 9-1-1 so the patient can be treated immediately.

We often can't imagine any good coming out of the worst of situations, but I see examples every single day that prove otherwise. With bad events such as a stroke, SCI, amputation, or TBI, it is hard to see good can come out of the worst circumstances. The worst thing in the world that happens to us often yields more good than bad. You are more resilient than you think and the power of your psychological immune system will prevail—if you learn how to let it; a victory yields happiness on the other side.

PART 2

PRINCIPLES OF THE HAPPINESS PERSPECTIVE IN HEALING

CHAPTER 4

THE HAPPINESS MUSCLE

Warning! Everything you think about happiness is wrong.

With over six hundred muscles in the human body, it is crazy to think I never learned about arguably the most important muscle we have during my studies in physical therapy school: *our happiness muscle!*

As a psychology major in my undergraduate work at Villanova University, the intricacies of the mind and how we think have always intrigued me. The brain, spinal cord, nerves, and manner in which they all communicate is truly miraculous. I remember learning about Daniel Gilbert and his work as a social psychologist. He is the author of *Stumbling on Happiness* and currently works at Harvard University. His work was highlighted in a podcast by Dr. Laurie Santos, a professor of psychology at Yale University and the host of *The Happiness Lab* podcast. As I investigated how the mind operates in relation to happiness, I started to see with much more clarity how many of my patients were able to unlock their own happiness. We can work to be happier, but we often put our time and efforts into the wrong things. Happiness needs to be an action and a change in habits. Our misconceptions of what we think happiness entails are completely distorted.

Dr. Santos discusses the work of Tim Wilson and Dan Gilbert and just how distorted our views of happiness really are. Let us begin with a concept by Dan Gilbert and his colleagues. The concept of mis-wanting is defined as "the act of being mistaken about what and how much you will like something in the future."[31] But why does this occur and why are we constantly mis-wanting?

Dr. Santos says there are four annoying features of the mind to explain this:

1. Our intuitions are just false. Our mind sometimes delivers information to us that is just wrong. A great concrete example of this is through vision. If you have not seen or heard of Shepard tables, they are a great example of how even when you know the answer and look at the tables over and over again, the intuition our vision is giving us that the tables are different sizes is wrong. The tables are in fact the same size.

2. Our minds do not think in terms of absolutes. We think in relative terms constantly comparing to a reference point. We are doing this and it messes up our judgment at hand. It is extremely hard to feel satisfied, especially when we are trying to fill our false intuitions. She describes how we have our own reference points and well as the

---

31   Daniel Gilbert and Timothy Wilson, *In Thinking and Feeling: The Role of Affect in Social Cognition* (Cambridge: Cambridge University Press, 2000), 8, 178-197.

reference point of others as a social comparison which sets us up for failure.

- A great example of this concept of reference points is by looking at one's salary. If we think in absolute terms, then making one hundred thousand dollars is better than making fifty thousand dollars. Right? What is interesting is being ABSOLUTELY better does not always make us feel better. It depends on our reference points. Unfortunately, the adage "misery loves company" has merit. There is an economic study describing this exact idea which examined the question below:
  - Would you rather make fifty thousand dollars a year and everyone else around you make twenty-five thousand dollars, OR would you rather make one hundred thousand dollars but everyone else around you is making two hundred thousand dollars? I was shocked to see about 50 percent of the people surveyed would give up half of their salary just to be doing better than other people. If we thought in terms of absolutes, it would make sense making one hundred thousand dollars is definitely better than making fifty thousand dollars; unfortunately, our minds love to trick us into thinking otherwise. [32]

3. The third reason we mis-want is because our minds habituate to things. Gilbert also described the concept of **hedonic adaptation** as the process of becoming accustomed to a positive or negative stimulus such the emotional effects of that stimulus are reduced over time. Tied

---

32   Ben Carlson, "A Wealth of Common Sense." *Perception Matters* (blog), November 13, 2014.

into this is the fact we don't even realize our minds are built to get used to this stuff. We think "happy things" we try to attain such as money, cars, and houses will last forever when, in fact, they do not. One quick way to combat this hedonistic adaptation is to spend money on experiences. We cannot adapt to new experiences and research shows experiences make us happier than buying "stuff." Lastly, when you spend money on experiences, you are less likely to make social comparisons.[33]

4. Lastly, Gilbert and colleagues came up with this idea of impact bias. They defined this as the tendency to overestimate the emotional impact of a future event both in terms of intensity and its duration. Mis-predicting intensity and duration of our own reactions prevents us from making decisions because of fear. He attributes this to two main reasons: *focalism*, defined as the tendency to think just about one event and forgetting everything else that can happen in our lives. The second reason is *immune neglect*, defined as the unawareness of our psychological immune system and the reality we are more resilient than we think. Bottom line: we underestimate ourselves.[34]

When we look at happiness with the framework Dr. Santos outlines, I believe the reference points are the most problematic. With social media, we have all these comparisons coming in for free and constantly flooding our biases. The advertisements that swamp our social media are something

---

33   Laurie Santos, "The Science of Well-Being" Yale University, Part One—Rethinking Awesome Stuff, video, 15:00.

34   Laurie Santos, "The Science of Well-Being," Yale University, Part One—Rethinking Awesome Stuff, video, 1:50.

we cannot control completely. We need to reset our reference points in our lives that Dr. Santos eludes to as well. I discuss some of the techniques in subsequent chapters as it relates to the framework of rehabilitation and recovery, but this is also applicable across different areas in our life.

Science and research tell us happiness correlation is attributable to many different aspects. Consider the work by Sonja Lyubomirsky. Her book highlights strategies backed by scientific research that can be used to increase happiness. She has done some really great work looking at what constitutes happiness including genes, life circumstances, and personal mindsets and actions. Her research is famous and most notably known for creating a pie chart to break down one's happiness.

Her findings show about **50 percent of one's happiness is in fact genetic**. Some people are more wired to be glass half-full type of people. This genetic set point makes up about 50 percent of the pie chart of happiness. What I found to be pretty remarkable (and echoed by Dr. Santos in her podcast) is **40 percent of our happiness can be attributed to our actions** and thoughts and about **10 percent can be attributed to life circumstances** and what happens to us, such as traumas or accidents one has to overcome in in his or her life. That means 40 percent of our happiness alone is under our control! We can work hard to be happier, but we have to be sure we are working toward the right things.[35]

---

35   Sonja Lyubomirsky, *The How of Happiness: A New Approach to Getting the Life You Want* (New York: The Penguin Press, 2008).

When I first set out on this journey of writing my book and conducting research, the four keys to unlocking one's happiness were purely anecdotal based on my experiences; however, the science and research I found also supports many of the characteristics I have witnessed to unlock happiness in trauma and beyond.

I was captivated by Robert Waldinger's TED Talk in 2015. Bob Waldinger is a professor of psychiatry and the fourth director for the last fifteen years of one of the longest studies conducted on human happiness. The eighty-year-old study is known as the Harvard Study of Adult Development. It began in 1938 and looks at the possible factors that lead to happiness and well-being. The study started looking at 268 Harvard sophomores and 456 boys from the poorest neighborhoods in Boston. They looked at health information as well as surveyed subjects every two years, asking them questions about their happiness.[36]

As years passed, they gathered more objective health information, such as blood tests and brain scans. This study included many interesting participants, such as President John F. Kennedy. The findings support the idea the keys to happiness do not involve achieving material things or working harder to achieve higher levels at work. Often, what people tend to sacrifice to collect material things and achieve more at work are the things that account for our true happiness. Waldinger says "the surprise was in our findings that one of the strongest predictors in staying healthy and happy

---

36 Robert Waldinger. "What Makes a Good Life? Lessons from the Longest Study on Happiness." November 2015, TED video, 10:52.

in your life was having good relationships with other people."[37] He asserts social connections are really good for us and it's not about the pure number of relationships but more their quality. These strong relationships are also protective for our health, including brain function and increased overall well-being. The bottom line is the happiest of people lean into relationships with family, friends, and the community.

Having this framework for happiness is paramount as you move forward in this journey. My expertise is in the human body as it relates to function and movement. I like to think of *happiness as a muscle*. For muscles to grow, a lot goes on. You cannot do the same exercise over and over with the same exact frequency and weight and expect to get stronger over time. If you enjoy running and are training for a marathon, you cannot merely run five miles in training and expect to run 26.2 miles with no problem. Muscle growth needs an approach that incorporates a variety of different facets to maximize their full potential. Stretching, good diet, hydration, and a balanced strengthening program are all important factors to consider for muscle growth and development. You might be able to get some strengthening from doing just resistance exercises, but to fully achieve our muscle's full potential, it has to be an approach that addresses multiple realms of muscle development.

Our happiness muscle needs this same approach. We cannot pick just one area to focus on. We have to constantly flex, stretch, and hydrate our happiness muscle on a daily basis.

37   Dr. Laurie Santos, "You Can Change," September 13, 2019, in *The Happiness Lab*, produced by Pushkin, podcast, MP3 audio, 21:54.

Some days our happiness muscles will feel really good—other days not so much. The important thing is to try to find different ways to help this muscle grow, develop, and thrive in this journey of life—regardless of the hand we're dealt.

One final thought to strengthen my argument of happiness being a muscle: as I see with my patients every single day, when we do not use our muscles, we lose them. Muscle atrophy is the literal wasting (thinning) or loss of muscle tissue. If we do not strengthen our happiness muscle, it will ultimately atrophy and start to waste away. Our "sadness muscle" will take over and it will be harder and harder to reverse the effects of our happiness muscle wasting. The beautiful thing about our muscles is no matter how weak or atrophied they get, with the right conditions and support, they CAN grow and get stronger. Happiness awaits us all and my hope, after reading this book, is you can start to *follow your smile* a little easier.

It is not enough to know the science when it comes to happiness. You have to go out there and do it. There is no quick fix or way to get to happiness. We have to be intentional to see changes **over time**. The framework for happiness I tackle is around physical trauma and recovery. You have to put the science into practice, and that is exactly what I have seen my happiest patients do following these four principles:

1. **Apathy into Altruism**
2. **Moment of Weakness versus Mentality of Weakness**
3. **Grief into Gratitude**
4. **Process versus Product**

You can make yourself happier. Your life circumstances are not as nearly as important as you think in deciding how happy you can be. The stories I share along with the science I have outlined will give you the tools to flex your happiness muscle with a little more confidence.

CHAPTER 5

APATHY INTO ALTRUISM

"What is the use of living, if it be not to strive for noble causes and to make this muddled world a better place for those who will live in it after we are gone?"

WINSTON CHURCHILL

Apathy is defined as lack of feeling or emotion.[38] This is common sentiment shared by the majority of my patients early on in the rehabilitation process. Interestingly, what makes the feeling of apathy so perplexing is it's the feeling of *not* feeling. Dr. Leon Seltzer is a clinical psychologist who says to "beware of apathy; it can be your worst enemy."[39] He shared this sentiment in an article posted in *Psychology Today*. Often when I first meet my patients, they lack a sense of relevance in

---

38 *Merriam-Webster*, s.v. "apathy (*n.*)," accessed October 7, 2020.

39 "The Curse of Apathy: Sources and Solutions," Psychology Today, accessed October 7, 2020.

their life since their injury. Seltzer says, "Without any com-
pelling emotion to direct your behavior, you just aren't suf-
ficiently stimulated to do much of anything."[40] My patients
are literally going through the motions and can no longer
see personal happiness or fulfillment is ever possible. They
do not see anything worth striving for when they have had
such a significant injury and their lives have been turned
upside down.

According to psychologists like Seltzer, strategies to help
with one's apathy have been explored. Getting sufficient
sleep, exercise, and avoiding alcohol may help decrease
apathy. Medications can also help. Cognitive therapy and
getting counseling are proven strategies as well. Having the
conversation with someone else can help to assist in unclog-
ging mental clutter and starting to see your purpose and
life through a new lens. While all of these avenues can be of
assistance, one specific path I have witnessed and am confident works is helping others. Altruism is defined as the
unselfish regard for or devotion to the welfare of others.[41]
Science supports altruistic behaviors and how they activate
reward centers in the brain.

One study in 2014 published in the journal of *Social Cognitive
and Affective Neuroscience* found engaging in such behaviors
activates the areas of the brain associated with the reward
system. Another interesting model shared in Seltzer's article
was the negative-state relief model. This model states human
beings have an innate drive to reduce any negative moods.

---

40   Ibid.

41   *Merriam-Webster*, s.v. "altruism (*n*.)," accessed October 4, 2020.

The premise is to engage in any mood-elevating behaviors, including helping others, to reduce your own negative affect and make you feel better.[42]

The idea of giving back, interacting, and helping others may seem a little counterintuitive when thinking about one's recovery after trauma; however, this may be one of the most impactful common threads I have noticed help my patients begin to shift their perspective and unlock their happiness. In my interview with Shannon, she highlighted the importance for her patients to give back and recognizes the power in doing so to help them start moving forward and find their new purpose. She went into the idea of our patients clinging to rehabilitation as a form of identity now, despite being months and years out of their injury, and treating rehabilitation as their full-time job.

She said, "My patients I have had that have finally accepted their injuries and have finally been like, you know what, I'm kind of where I am and I need to find purpose in life and they get a job or volunteer. I feel like those people are the ones that find their happiness because they are giving back and they are not just looking to try to improve themselves but help others."[43]

As far as my own patients, one particular patient of mine speaks to just how powerful giving back and finding a community to surround yourself with can be in beginning to turn

---

42   "Negative-State Relief Model," Psychology Research and Reference, accessed April 23, 2020.

43   Shannon Motisi, conversation with author, April 15, 2020.

the key in the direction of happiness. I run the amputee support group with a colleague and friend, Heather. We meet monthly at the rehabilitation hospital where I work. I first met the patient at a meeting when he was still early in the recovery process. He had lost his leg below the knee due to diabetes and vascular issues. The amputation occurred two weeks earlier, when I first met him, and he was now in inpatient care at Kessler, learning how to move around in his wheelchair and perform normal, everyday activities, commonly referred to as Activities of Daily Living or ADLs. His incision still needed to heal, so it would be a few more weeks before he would get his prosthesis and begin learning how to use it.

When I met him that evening at the support group, he was sitting in his wheelchair, slouched over, quiet, and reserved. His body language was the epitome of apathy. During the hour and half support group meeting, he may have said five words. Every time I glanced at him, he was staring out at the wall or down at the table in front of him. His very supportive wife was keenly listening to every word the members of the group were sharing. I introduced myself at the end of the meeting, thanked them both for coming, and provided my information so they could reach out to me if they had any questions.

As his apathy lingered with me that night, I found myself tossing and turning in bed until I was finally able to sleep. He was eventually discharged from the acute rehabilitation part of the hospital and deemed ready to go home because he was safe with the ADLs previously mentioned. A few weeks later, I was evaluating him for his outpatient therapy with me. His leg healed beautifully and before coming to see me, he received his prosthesis from his prosthetist. After my one hour initial evaluation with him seated in his wheelchair, I began to see glimpses of happiness come to the surface in the narrative he was painting since returning home from the hospital.

Over the course of the next two months, he was able to put his leg on independently, go from walking into therapy with a rolling walker to being able to use only a cane, and ascending and descending a flight of stairs. His apathy I witnessed just three months earlier slowly began to turn into enthusiasm and a new appreciation on life. Whether he knew it or not, he was beginning to turn the key in the direction of unlocking his own happiness perspective. The ultimate transformative moment occurred when he and his wife came to the support group again. He walked in with his head up high and the overall juxtaposition from when I first met him was truly uplifting. The most inspirational moment was him answering questions of the other members of the group about his journey to help them try and understand what to expect. I could not shut him up if I tried; his metamorphosis would not be possible if he remained isolated and alone.

Recovery after trauma can be a very lonely process, but as highlighted earlier, it does not have to be. Research asserts loneliness can make you sicker than smoking cigarettes and being part of a supportive community can increase your life expectancy. Dr. Lissa Rankin highlights this exact notion in her book *Mind Over Medicine*.[44] Roseto, Pennsylvania in 1961

44   Lissa Rankin, *Mind Over Medicine: Scientific Proof that You Can Heal Yourself* (Carlsbad: Hay House, Inc., 2013).

is living proof of the power of being part of something bigger than oneself. Dr. Stewart Wolf, a professor at the University of Oklahoma School of Medicine, bought a summer home in the Poconos, not far away.

This little town of Roseto was of particular interest to Dr. Wolf because heart disease seemed far less prevalent there than in the adjoining towns. After doing some research and digging deeper, Dr. Wolf found men in neighboring cities of Roseto had heart attack rates on par with the national average at the time, which was the number one cause of death in men under sixty-five. Contrary to neighboring cities, Roseto's heart attack rate was half the national average. What is more interesting is there was no suicide, alcoholism, drug addiction, and very little crime recorded among these patients. They even looked at peptic ulcers in these patients who didn't have any of those either. These particular people were dying of old age—and that's it![45]

After interviewing two-thirds of the adult population, it was determined diet and physical activity were not the best practices and 41 percent of their calories came from fat. Investigation began to look at genetics by looking at the cousins and relatives scattered around; however, these relatives were no healthier than average so that theory was out the window. After his interviews and research, Dr. Wolf concluded the tight-knit community was a better predictor of heart health than cholesterol levels or tobacco use. Fast-forward twenty years and the people of Roseto started to disband and

---

45 Malcolm Gladwell, *Outliers: The Story of Success* (New York: Little, Brown, & Company, 2008).

younger generations went off to study. They brought back new ideas, dreams, and new people to marry. By the end of the 1970s, the number of fatal heart attacks in Roseto had increased to the national average. In Dr. Rankin's book, she explains how human beings nourish one another—and our happiness muscle.

A Harvard study examined the lives of almost three thousand senior citizens. Those who were more social, going out to dinners, movies, playing cards, and engaging in such behaviors outlived their peers by an average of three years. As I continue to notice in my career, even the degree of social support you experience affects the likelihood of cure. A University of California, San Francisco, study published in the *Journal of Clinical Oncology* looked at the social networks of nearly three thousand nurses with breast cancer. This particular study found the women who went through cancer alone were four times more likely to die from their disease than those with ten or more friends supporting their journey.[46]

The more I see my patients participate in community events, volunteering, and support groups, the happier they are. Altruistic behaviors and being part of something bigger than oneself may prove to be as important as exercise when it comes to predicting outcomes in therapy and even life expectancy. If I am working with a patient who does everything they are supposed to do with regards to their rehabilitation

---

46   Candyce H. Kroenke et al., "Social Networks, Social Support, and Survival after Breast Cancer Diagnosis" *Journal of Clinical Oncology* 24, no.7 (March 1, 2006): 1105 -1111.

process, but are alone and relatively have a sense of apathy, often times they fall into some sort of depression.

In an interview with Sean O'Donnell, he recognizes the importance of giving back and the impact it has had on his recovery; he carries with him in his daily mindset to give back and help others. I learned about Sean from a social media post from the Villanova community. Sean suffered a spinal cord injury, leaving him paralyzed from his waist down when he was seventeen years old. He was hit by a car in 1995 while riding his motorcycle. Since then, he has become a successful product manager, computer engineer, motivational speaker, writer, and pilot. Sean did his rehabilitation in Philadelphia at Magee Rehabilitation. Of all the things Sean has accomplished over the past twenty-five years since his injury, he states "my proudest personal achievement is enabling other people with disabilities to achieve their dreams."[47]

Sean was obsessed with flying growing up, according to his interview with the *Philadelphia Inquirer*, and was a huge *Top Gun* fan. Years after his spinal cord injury, O'Donnell came across Able Flight, a nonprofit founded in 2006. The mission of this organization connects people with disabilities to pilot training programs. Sean earned his license through Able Flight and now mentors other pilots. During my interview with Sean, I learned of a project he was involved in with a few of his old friends. The collaboration, entitled *Rise Like the Phoenix*, highlights stories of people who have suffered some form of life-changing accidents or health challenges.

---

47   Sean O'Donnell, conversation with author, March 3, 2020.

The purpose of his book speaks to the importance of this chapter's message: helping others and giving back.

I wrapped up my interview with Sean by asking him one last question: "What is your definition of happiness?"

He stated, "I have locked it (happiness) down to one thing and it's the same thing I say to everyone when they are feeling sad or down." He continued, "When someone usually tells me they are feeling bad, I ask them, *who have you helped today?* You are feeling depressed or sad? Who have you helped today? Get out there and help somebody and, in turn, you will help yourself. If you want to help yourself, go help somebody else. It gives you perspective, it gives you reward, and it's far more valuable than any dollar you will ever earn. I think it's the ultimate lead to happiness."[48]

As I try to explain to my patients, when it comes to giving back and socializing, there is no cookie-cutter recipe to do so. The important thing to understand is you are not alone and there are people out there who have similar experiences and traumas. The quicker my patients realize this, the quicker they can tap into their new purpose and move forward. As Dr. Wolf revealed with the Roseto community, I have also noticed with my patients that individuals who are surrounded by a supportive community and find ways to give back helps to relax the body. This relaxation translates into positive effects on the body's physiology.

---

48   Sean O'Donnell, conversation with author, March 3, 2020.

My patients who are able to turn their apathy into altruism are the ones I have seen make the biggest steps in their recovery. I have seen the smallest altruistic behaviors have lasting impacts for both the helper and person being helped. It snowballs into more acts of altruism, which is exactly what this world needs more of, in recovery and beyond. If you told me helping others would be a key in recovery for my patients when I first started my career as a physical therapist, I would be skeptical, too. Reflecting over the past few years made me realize just how important *turning your apathy into altruism is.*

What are some ways you can help others to help you unlock your own happiness?

CHAPTER 6

MOMENT OF WEAKNESS VERSUS MINDSET OF WEAKNESS

———

"Our greatest weakness lies in giving up. The most certain way to succeed is always to try just one more time."

THOMAS EDISON

Throughout any phase of recovery I see my patients going through, it is inevitable to have moments of wanting to give up completely. The patients who I have seen unlock their happiness perspective all have a common thread as they navigate through their recovery. Devon Still was a guest on the *School of Greatness* podcast. Devon is a professional athlete, author, motivational speaker, and advocate for childhood cancer awareness. Along with his collegiate and professional football accolades, he is more recently known for helping his daughter fight cancer. In this particular episode, he discussed his journey throughout each of these stages of his life. His main message and mission is to put as much positivity in this world as possible and let people know whatever they are going through or facing, it can be overcome. I always try and share the same narrative with my patients. I encourage them to be vulnerable and let them know it is okay to not be okay—for moments.

Devon touches on this exact message. I find myself doing it more and more as I learn and grow in my career. Devon was discussing how, when his daughter first was diagnosed with cancer, he felt it was his fault. He felt deep down he could have done something differently or could have provided for her in a better way so she would not have been diagnosed. He speaks to the importance and lessons he learned during this time and how he was able to be vulnerable and understand it was not his fault. It will be a team effort and there will be days you want to give up, but you will make it through. *Allow yourself to have those weak moments, but don't allow it to snowball into a weak mindset.*[49]

Consider Thomas Edison's work with the light bulb. In the period from 1878 to 1880, Edison and his associates worked on at least three thousand different theories to develop an efficient incandescent lamp. He tested thousands and thousands of materials to use for the filament. He began to test the carbonized filaments of every plant imaginable and, despite the work being extremely tedious and demanding, he always

---

49   Lewis Howes, "Embrace Your Struggle with Devon Still," February 27, 2019, in *The School of Greatness* podcast, MP3 audio, 44:45.

recognized the importance of hard work and determination. He has said, "Before I got through, I tested no fewer than six thousand vegetable growths and ransacked the world for the most suitable filament material." Edison's perseverance epitomizes how moments of failure are more than okay; however, allowing them to turn into a mentality is the real kryptonite of progress.

Little did I know, when my soccer career came to a screeching halt (temporarily), I would be heeding my own advice based on lessons I have learned from the patients I have treated twenty years later. Let me wind back the clock to my freshman year in college. It was August of 2004 and the Villanova men's soccer team was preparing for a new campaign. I did not carry some of the credentials as some of the other freshman going into preseason, and to be fair, my name was not on the radar of most of the major Division I soccer schools in the recruiting process. I earned entry into Villanova University on my academic merit and was given the chance to make the roster that summer. Preseason started with a grueling fitness test and I knew I had to prepare in the months leading up to it to make sure I would impress the coaching staff.

I felt great during the fitness test and passed it with flying colors. I felt like I was competing in all the practices and never for a second thought I would not make the final squad. The business of paring a roster down to manageable size is seldom easy, but I honestly felt I deserved to be on the team based on how the three weeks of preseason went. At our last practice, on Villanova's West campus, the team was walking off the pitch. As I was ready to head off, my coach at the time called me over.

"Hey coach, what's up?" I said as I approached him.

"How you feeling?" He replied.

"Honestly, I feel really good and felt like I had a strong few weeks."

"No easy way to tell you this, but unfortunately, I will not be able to offer you a spot on the team."

My emotions immediately boiled up to the back of my throat and I could not get a word out. All I remember was asking what I could have done better or differently and got defensive based on his decision. It is amazing how our mind and body automatically go into defense mode.

What followed was a vigorous exploration of how I was going to let those who loved me know what had just happened. I walked away from the coach, exacerbated physically and emotionally, laid on my back, stared up at the predawn summer sky and just cried. Soccer was my identity. Ever since I could remember, I was playing soccer. My parents made many sacrifices, especially my mom. She dutifully took me to practices multiple times a week or spent weekends on major holidays at soccer tournaments, missing family events; I did not know how to tell my family I had just been cut from the team. I did not want to disappoint them and that's exactly what I felt I did. After breaking the news to them, I immediately realized there was no time for self-pity.

I funneled my energy into keeping my dream alive. I worked out on my own and made sure I stayed in the best physical shape. I kept annoying coach during the season and kept emailing him and showing up at all the games to let him know I was really interested. Fast-forward a few months and when I got out there in the first game of the spring, I felt confident I was where I was supposed to be. By the close of the 2005 season, I was a regular and appeared in fourteen games, including multiple starting assignments, ultimately leading to a full scholarship by my senior year. The lessons, friendships, and experiences that followed as a direct result of what the beautiful game has taught me would have never happened if I had let one moment of weakness turn into a mindset of weakness.

I knew what I could do. I had to believe in myself and know what I was capable of doing. Sometimes we have to be our own cheerleader. Sometimes we have to want it bad enough to try and really put ourselves out there and do the best we can—then see where we land. Another valuable lesson I learned here is the fact I did not want to have any regrets. I mentioned in my introduction most people regret so much in their life. If I did not try again during spring season, I would have regretted it for the rest of my life. Deep down, I knew I did not want to walk away from the game I loved so much. If it did not work out, I would have been okay with the end result knowing I tried.

I have always wondered why some of my patients have been able to improve more drastically and quickly while others almost seemed not interested at all and showed only marginal signs of improvement. How can we limit the duration we have from these moments of weakness and not let them fester? As I continued to investigate and research this question, I have come to the conclusion grit is an instrumental characteristic to possess. The scientific research is clear experiencing trauma without control can be debilitating. I see it every day.

In Angela Duckworth's exploration of grit, she highlights the secret to outstanding achievement is a special blend of passion and persistence. My colleague and good friend, Heather, gave me a copy of this amazing book called *Grit*. This book has helped me so much in shaping my perspective on life. Additionally, how I treat my patients. I used to think hope was the answer, but after doing some research, I believe now it has to be more. Duckworth makes it very clear while hope offers some kind of reprieve from the current situation one is in, "the onus is on the universe to make things better."[50]

Grit, she contends, depends on a different kind of hope. We do not have to wait for the universe to make things better. Grit rests on the expectation our own efforts can improve our future. When my patients have these moments of weakness, the ones who can "snap out of it" the quickest tend to tell themselves through their direct actions and choices, they have the resolve to make tomorrow better. Some of my patients believe, deep down, they can change. Duckworth classifies these individuals as growth-oriented people.[51] Given the right opportunity and support, and if they try hard enough, they will improve. Fixed mindset individuals are my patients who cling on to the fact they will never improve, no matter what they do. It is important to note even

---

50   Angela Duckworth, *Grit* (New York: Scribner, 2016), 169.

51   Duckworth, *Grit*, 180.

if someone is considered more of a fixed-minded individual, there are avenues for change. Cognitive behavioral therapy helps patients think more objectively and behave in healthier ways and is a powerful intervention to help individuals practice interpreting what happens to them and respond with a positive outlook.

In my interview with Eric LeGrand, I asked him how he limits these moments of weakness to minimize the risk of slipping into a prolonged mentality of weakness. I have come to know Eric over the past few years through his rehabilitation process and he is truly an inspiration and epitomizes the meaning of grit.

When I asked him about how he is able to get through those low points and moments when he feels like he is having a bad day, he says, "You have to look at things and have the perspective on life that okay, you may be frustrated now, but you know it could be a lot worse off than what you are. Although everything feels like things may be going the wrong way, you can still push through and you can still make it through if you look at the little things that actually matter in your life and the people that you have. That is how I get through my every day."[52]

Regardless of the struggles you might be going through, the point is you can change your internal dialogue. With repeated practice, guidance, and gratitude, you can change the way you think, feel, and heal. I have seen it firsthand from my patients with the way they believe so deeply and the

---

52   Eric LeGrand, conversation with author, March 27, 2020.

grit they demonstrate on a daily basis. Duckworth recounts a story of a woman named Rhonda who reached out to her, recommending a change to her grit scale. Duckworth heeded the recommendation and I am happy she did.

The grit scale used to say, "Setbacks don't discourage me."

Rhonda said, "That makes no sense. I mean, who doesn't get discouraged by setbacks? I certainly do. I think it should say, 'Setbacks don't discourage me for long. I get back on my feet.'"[53]

My patients are confronted with this option almost every single day throughout recovery. There are countless times when they want to give up and not try anymore, and it honestly might be easier for them. I always tell my patients to keep going and keep pushing forward when they are having moments of weakness. I am not asking them to do something I haven't done myself, which is to persevere even amidst setbacks, because one never knows when success may come. Lastly, as a physical therapist, I make sure I listen to my patients. Part of what I do is to offer instruction and motivation so they are able to take the moments of weakness they have and turn them into positive driving points.

Jay Wright has been Villanova University's men's basketball coach since 2001. He has won two national championships and, in 2016, won the Naismith College Basketball Coach of the Year award. In his book, *Attitude*, he highlights how to cultivate a winning mindset on and off the court. He

---

53   Angela Duckworth, *Grit* (New York: Scribner, 2016), 194.

asserts, "Offering instruction for improvement is necessary, of course, but it never hurts to solicit input...try asking what they think could be done better. Those conversations are often illuminating."[54]

My grittiest patients are the ones who unlock their happiness the quickest. They are motivated and genuinely believe their actions and thoughts can better their current situation. Regardless of the situation they may be in, they are fighting for a better tomorrow for themselves. For me, *grit is the antidote to preventing moments of weakness from spiraling into a mentality of weakness.*

54   Jay Wright, *Attitude: Develop a Winning Mindset on and off the Court* (New York: Ballentine Books, 2017), 197.

CHAPTER 7

GRIEF INTO GRATITUDE

Gratitude: "Trade your expectations
for appreciation and your whole life
will change in that moment."

TONY ROBBINS

"How can I show any appreciation for having my leg amputated?"

This question and sentiment is a common one early in the recovery process for most of my patients. When confronting trauma and grief, having any sense of gratitude or appreciation seems impossible. It takes time and seeing others in the therapy gym to change their perspectives. I cannot tell you how many times I have treated a below-knee amputee and they have expressed gratitude once they see a patient learning how to use an above-knee prosthesis and the challenges that come with it.

Every day my patients see just how bad a stroke, brain injury, or amputation can really be. These patients express how thankful they are they *only* lost their leg below their knee versus above. They are thankful in their ability to use an arm versus both an arm and a leg, or can only walk with a walker versus being stuck in a wheelchair. From my experiences and interactions with my patients, my lens of gratitude is constantly being refocused. I realized just how important the transition from grief to gratitude is in my patients' recovery. I investigate the link between the two in this chapter and how it assists in their overall happiness in their recovery.

Grief is a reaction to loss. "The grief associated with death is familiar to most of us, but we grieve a wide variety of losses throughout our lives: traumatic experiences, divorce, relocation, loss of health and mobility are only some examples. Grief is often expressed by feelings such as anger, guilt, sadness, or loneliness. But grief affects us in other ways as well—spiritually, behaviorally, physically, and cognitively."[55]

I have noticed grief is very personal and in no way is it a one-shoe-fits-all type of timeline. It is important to note not everyone experiences all five stages and there is no set time-table for each stage. My patients respond to grief after injury in a variety of different ways, including crying, anger, and withdrawal. Elisabeth Kubler-Ross was a psychiatrist who established the Kubler-Ross model and wrote in her book grief could be divided into five stages:

---

55   "Grief," Hospice Foundation of America, accessed May 23, 2020.

1. Denial
2. Anger
3. Bargaining
4. Depression
5. Acceptance

What I have noticed with my patients is once they accept their injuries, they understand what they mean in their lives now and how to better move forward. This particular stage is not always a positive or uplifting stage. They may have not moved past the grief or loss completely, but they start to pivot in a positive direction. Treatment for grief varies from patient to patient and can include a myriad of options, including cognitive behavior therapy and medically-assisted therapy (medications to assist with symptoms of grieving processes). One thing I have noticed that helps my patients in their grieving process is their faith. I have watched people with unbelievable challenges in their physical situations, personal life, and their family life. Often I think to myself, how in the world can this person get through this?

I interviewed Bonnie Evans, the CEO of Kessler Institute of Rehabilitation in West Orange, New Jersey. She says one key ingredient she noticed in her experiences in overcoming grief as it relates to physical trauma and beyond is for patients to have a foundation in faith. She says, "The fact that patients have a foundation of faith already gives them a strength and wisdom and understanding that allows them to unlock their happiness."[56] I asked about the patients who do not have faith. She responded by saying, "Because of the people they

---

56   Bonnie Evans, conversation with author, May 12, 2020.

interacted with who did (have faith), that development of faith, and it does not have to be a faith in the God that I know, but a faith in a being or in a universe that is higher and outside yourself, they were also able to accept their situation much quicker."[57] I share Bonnie's sentiment and know during the grieving stages after a life-changing injury, those with some sort of foundation in faith have been able to lean into it and keep them from falling over the edge.

The word gratitude is derived from the Latin word gratia, which means grace, graciousness, or gratefulness.[58] At its most basic sense, gratitude is a thankful appreciation for what an individual receives and can be either material or intangible. Researchers in Positive Psychology have found gratitude and happiness are always strongly correlated. Gratitude moves people to experience more positive emotions. As soon as my patients tap into this particular practice, I see them start to enjoy good experiences, better their health, face adversity, and start to really make a shift in their recovery. There are three main ways people can express their gratitude: by being gracious of their past, present, or for what's to come.[59]

Recent evidence suggests a promising approach to complement psychological counseling with additional activities that are not too taxing for clients but yield high results.

57   Ibid.

58   "Giving Thanks Can Make You Happier," Harvard Health Publishing. Harvard Medical School, accessed May 20, 2020.

59   "The Science and Research on Gratitude and Happiness," Positive Psychology, accessed May 15, 2020.

Additionally, the reality of polypharmacy—the simultaneous use of multiple drugs to treat a single condition—in the medical world is prevalent. If gratitude can offer such powerful and therapeutic effects on the body, it is worth investigating to see if this relatively easy tool can help with potentially eliminating some medications on which so many patients rely.

As I began to investigate the impact of gratitude on the human body, I found most research studies on gratitude have been conducted with well-functioning people. I wanted to explore if gratitude is beneficial for people who struggle with physical and mental health concerns. In a study conducted by Dr. Joel Wong and Dr. Joshua Brown involving nearly three hundred adults, they found gratitude to be a powerful tool in managing anxiety and depression.

The study consisted of three groups. All the groups received counseling services; however, the first group was also instructed to write one letter of gratitude to another person each week for three weeks. The second group was asked to write about their deepest thoughts and feelings about negative experiences. The last group did not do any writing activity. They found the group who wrote gratitude letters reported significantly better mental health even twelve weeks after their writing exercise ended. The study did not stop there. The authors investigated and wanted to explore how gratitude might actually work on our minds and bodies.[60]

---

60 Joel Y. Wong et al., "Does Gratitude Writing Improve the Mental Health of Psychotherapy Clients? Evidence from a Randomized Controlled Trial," *Psychotherapy Research* 28, no. 2 (2016): 192-202.

Those in the gratitude writing group used a higher percentage of positive emotion words and lower proportion of negative emotion words than those in the other writing group. The lack of negative emotion words explained the mental health gap between the gratitude writing group and the other writing group. The investigators assert when one's attention is shifted away from toxic emotions, such as depression, guilt, or resentment, it translates into better mental and physical health. The second layer they tapped into was of particular interest to me. They found gratitude helps even if you do not share it. When the study started, the participants in the group who wrote gratitude letters were not required to send to their intended recipient. Only 23 percent of the participants ended up delivering them. I found it interesting that the mental health benefits of just writing the letter was not dependent on actually sending it.[61]

This finding made me think about the power of the different ways I personally try and implement practices of gratitude and have found it helps to start my day on the right note. In the entrance of my apartment, I have a key holder with a small blackboard to write on and every morning (or most mornings), I try to write one thing I am grateful for before I leave for work. It gets me to actively think about and reflect on what I do have and helps to elicit positive sentiments versus negative ones. It is a personal activity I now know sows amazing changes in my mindset. Gratitude doesn't have to be saved for the big things in life; the habit of being grateful starts with appreciating every good thing in life and recognizing there is nothing too small for you to be thankful for.

---

61   Ibid.

Some ways my patients have put this into practice that may be a helpful tool for you is to write a thank you note, keep a journal, or pick a set time every week to actually count your blessings. Having a set time in your schedule can be a powerful tool to practice gratitude.

The last two findings of the study reported gratitude's benefits can take time. There was not a difference in mental health levels one week after the end of the writing activities, but the gratitude writing group reported better mental health than the other groups four weeks after the writing; this difference in mental health became even larger twelve weeks after the conclusion of the study.[62] The bottom line is not to get discouraged if you don't magically feel better after writing one letter. The benefits of this practice may take time to actually manifest themselves. It is a process and a journey that requires patience.

This crucial insight got me thinking. We rush through life. In David's Steindl-Rast's TED Talk, he discusses the importance of patience in gratitude. David is a monk and interfaith scholar. In his talk, he says we need to do a better job of creating stop signs in our lives which will allow us to enjoy the moments and be thankful for the opportunities. The key is "to stop, look, and go."[63] This method will help us live in gratitude consistently and not just for moments. We miss the opportunities in our life because we do not stop. At best, we yield and never can appreciate the small moments and

---

62 Ibid.

63 David Steindl-Rast, "Want to be Happy? Be Grateful." June 2013, TED video, 5:45.

victories in our lives. I personally have learned to add more stop signs in my life, look both ways, and move forward with gratitude.

It often takes time for my patients to start practicing any sense of gratitude during their recovery. What I continue to notice as they start expressing gratitude and shifting their perspective is their recovery also starts pivoting in the right direction.

One particular patient of mine spoke to the moment she was able to make her pivot from grief into gratitude (it pains me to write the next sentence being a Villanova University graduate, but for the sake of happiness and helping others, I will put my Nova Nation roots to the side). My patient, Madeline Niebanck (Maddi), graduated from Georgetown University. Her lens of gratitude shifted early in her recovery and is the catalyst for how well she progressed since her stroke. I asked her how she shifted her mindset so early in recovery. She talks about living the process of going through rehabilitation and how there was one moment that set the tone for her moving forward. While she was in acute inpatient rehabilitation for five weeks, she had time between therapies. During her down time, visitors would come and go to help pass the time she was not working in the gym. On a walk with her brother, she was going up and down the hallway when she became fatigued and needed a seat.

"At the time I was only able to walk twenty feet before needing to sit down in the wheelchair. There was this moment when I was walking with my ace wrap (to keep my foot up) and my quad cane (for balance) and I was like, I hate my life...this is terrible." She is able to say this with laughter now. "We had stopped in front of another person's room and when I glanced over, I noticed a patient who was completely paralyzed and clearly could not even do anything at all near what I was doing. I had this moment where I said to myself, oh shit—there are people who would do anything to be able to just stand up."[64] Later in the conversation, Maddi explained how prior to this moment, the narrative she was telling herself was one of grief and sense of feeling sorry for herself and complaining she was no longer able to do what she could do before. In that very moment, she changed her grief into gratitude. She literally stopped walking and, while seated, shifted the narrative and said, "Look at me. I can stand up. I can stand up and take a step. Yes, I can only walk twenty feet before I need to take a break, but I can do that. That is an overlooked thing where you forget how amazing that is."[65]

When I first started interviewing happiness perspective paragons, most of them shared how seeing someone's situation worse than theirs helped them make the pivot to gratitude. Like Maddi's story, many of my patients have these moments that help them start to shift their perspectives. I started to wonder and ask myself why do we have to see someone in a bleak situation to make that shift? As I continued interviewing patients who have unlocked their happiness, I realized we should not base our gratitude on circumstances in our lives because they can change in a heartbeat. David Steindl-Rast's message is happiness is born from gratitude. An inspiring lesson in slowing down, looking where you're going, and

---

64 Madeline Niebanck, conversation with author, March 26, 2020.

65 Ibid.

above all, being grateful. Whether it takes seeing someone worse off than us or not, turning grief into gratitude is one of the most integral ways in recovering from trauma. You can cultivate a sense of appreciation and you can teach yourself to be thankful. As you approach your first stop sign and begin to move forward, what are you thankful for?

CHAPTER 8

PROCESS VERSUS PRODUCT

———

"A systems-first mentality provides the antidote. When you fall in love with the process rather than the product, you don't have to wait to give yourself permission to be happy."

JAMES CLEAR

"How long will it be before I am able to do things like I used to before my injury?"

I am asked this question multiple times a week. Most of the time it is my patient. Other times it is a family member or caregiver asking for their loved one. Having no insight into the rehabilitation process after a neurological injury, this is a valid question, but before giving away how I will typically answer them, let's explore the core principle in this chapter of process over product.

I was listening to a podcast hosted by Ed Mylett. He is a prominent entrepreneur and the host of *The Ed Mylett Show*. He showcases the greatest peak performers across all industries, sharing their journey, knowledge, and thoughts about leadership. His main goal is to inspire, through practical steps, and help his audience become the best versions of themselves. He interviewed Inky Johnson on one of his podcasts, entitled *The Winning Mentality*. I had never heard of Inky before and I was inspired when he started talking about this idea of "process over product" after his career-ending injury.[66] His drive, not only in his recovery, but in his daily life moving forward struck a chord with me and I want to explore deeper. The concept of eliminating the final product of his recovery and focusing more on the journey and process was one of the key takeaways. My patients who unlock their happiness echo the same sentiments about trusting the **process versus focusing on the final product.**

September 9, 2006 started as a normal college football game in Neyland Stadium at the University of Tennessee for Inky. The game changed everything after a routine tackle turned into a life-threatening injury and nothing has been normal for him since. Inky was born in Atlanta in 1986 and from an early age, he always had a dream to play professional football. Unfortunately (or fortunately), his dream never came to fruition. He suffered a brachial plexus injury during his junior year that would leave his right arm completely paralyzed.

---

66   Ed Mylett, "Perspective Drives Performance with Inky Johnson," February 5, 2020, in *The Ed Mylett Show*, podcast, MP3 audio, 33:30.

In his podcast, he discusses his journey. He woke up from his injury and his initial reaction was his career was not over. He thought he could go to rehab and get back on the field. His doubt really set in and he was just a few games away from entering the NFL draft and living out his dream. From early on in his recovery, he was able to eliminate the end result of his recovery, which allowed him to walk into the situation with a concrete mentality. He had the ability to start his journey of recovery, stay focused, and stay the course without any guarantee of the end result. He asserts it should be driven by one's integrity and character.[67] To take it one step further, when we start anything new in our lives with a strong focus on the end result, disappointment, anxiety, and regret manifests if we fail to reach our destination.

He goes on to discuss different driving forces in his life who helped strengthen his loyalty: his coaches, teammates, teachers, family, and people who supported him along the way. It is important to have driving forces that are not superficial or materialistic. If we have driving forces every single day of our lives that are of value, like our children, work, spouse, the people who helped you get to a certain point in your life, and so on, you are better equipped to handle struggle and adversity. Another key point Inky touches upon is this notion of perspective driving performance. The moment we shift our perspective and embrace it, it changes not only us but everyone and everything connected to us. Adversity can now be viewed as an opportunity.

---

67   Ed Mylett, "Perspective Drives Performance with Inky Johnson," February 5, 2020, in *The Ed Mylett Show*, podcast, MP3 audio, 35:10.

One example that comes to mind and bears a striking resemblance is a young patient of mine: Maddi, who I introduced in the last chapter. Her story is a little unique because she knew she was going into surgery to try and fix what is called an arteriovenous malformation (AVM). An AVM is a tangle of abnormal blood vessels connecting arteries and veins in the brain and is essentially not formed properly; most of the time from birth. It can go undetected for the duration of someone's life and nothing can happen, but she had migraines since she could remember. As she got older, the frequency and intensity of her migraines reached a point she was unable to tolerate any longer. After significant deliberation, she decided it was time to try and fix the malformation. Unfortunately, she ended up having a stroke which resulted in her having one side of her body paralyzed.

During my interview with Maddi, she reflected on the notion of the process versus focusing on the goal or end product. She said, "Here's the thing, and I don't think a lot of people want to hear this, but it's a lifelong process. You are not just going to magically get better after having a stroke…it is just going to be a constant lifelong process that I have to work on." I recognize getting to this perspective and arriving at this realization varies from person to person and is not an easy mindset to attain. We all have goals we want to achieve and setting these goals is instrumental in getting where we want to go. I am not saying we should not be setting goals, but it is more important to focus on the actual process and the systems one uses to get there. Maddi summed it up best toward the end of my interview with her when she said, "You have to literally fall in love with the process."[68]

I realized this transcended the realm of recovery and injury in the healthcare domain, as I'd seen in my own life. Running has been an integral part of my life—through the game of soccer and beyond. I have settled into a career I love. I was driven to achieve my entire life. I was driven to be great in sports, and when sports were over, to be great in physical therapy school, which worked. I achieved great results playing division I Big East soccer at Villanova University and climbing the ranks in my job to clinical manager.

I did not know how to turn it off. I was always striving for bigger and better while focusing on the achievements and it was never enough. I always thought accomplishing these things would lead to happiness, but for whatever reason, I was left feeling this sort of emptiness with no real ending in sight. Over the past few years, I have learned through a variety of platforms and experiences; running is one of them. I am a big believer in challenging yourself to grow. With running, I find I get to challenge myself. Inky Johnson's notion of living in the moment and trying not to think about the future or the past is epitomized in running—most notably when running a marathon.

November 6, 2016 was a picture-perfect crisp fall day. Fifty thousand runners lined up to start the New York City Marathon on the foot of the Verrazzano-Narrows Bridge in Staten Island. I had never thought of the bridge as narrow

---

68   Madeline Niebanck, conversation with author, March 26, 2020.

until all those people were on there. Interestingly enough, it is the longest suspension bridge in North America and one that also prohibits running on all other days of the year. I was so happy to be on the upper level of the bridge as I heard stories of people getting peed on when on the lower level.

The cannon sounded and as I was trying not to trip on my fellow runners, I took in the view to my left of the Manhattan skyline. Miles two through thirteen are all through vastly different neighborhoods, including Bay Ridge, Sunset Park, Williamsburg, Fort Green, and the Bedford-Stuyvesant sections of Brooklyn. The halfway point of the run leads to the Pulaski Bridge, which connects Brooklyn and Queens and is named for a Polish hero of the American Revolution. The next two miles navigate runners through Queens (home of my New York Mets) and ultimately to Manhattan, which was the most memorable point of the race for me. At mile sixteen, you quite literally go up and away. The incline on the Verrazzano-Narrows Bridge back at mile one was actually longer than of the Fifty-Ninth Street Bridge, but I barely noticed it.

It was a bright beautiful day, yet I felt like I was in a darkened tunnel with how quiet it was on the incline. There was no one around; only my fellow marathoners' footsteps. As I reached the summit, I felt my muscles transitioning from contracting to coasting as I let the decline facilitate and guide my legs. There was a faint sound up ahead that gradually got louder and louder, ultimately turning into a rising roar. In my head, I knew my parents and brother as well as my friend were waiting for me along with the swarms of well-wishers welcoming us to Manhattan. Ten miles to go and up First Avenue I went through East Harlem and ultimately to the Willis Avenue Bridge, which connects Manhattan to the Bronx and back over the Madison Avenue Bridge, which carries runners back into Manhattan. Down Fifth Avenue, I went for five more miles along the East side of Central Park to the twenty-fifth mile. I made my last right turn onto Central Park South for a straight half-mile shot toward the finish line, enjoying every step during the three-hour and forty-two minute process.

For me, running embodies living in the moment and not dwelling on the things you cannot control. This really is the greatest gift running has given to me. My friend's sister asked me what I think about when I run, and after pondering about it for a few seconds, I do not think it was the answer she was looking for: nothing! It is the one time of the day my mind is at peace and I am not multi-tasking. I am not saying running is easy; at times it's absolutely miserable, but it forces me to look inward and to challenge and focus on the process. Running is about being present and experiencing the moment, which is such an important mindset and perspective to have in this crazy and nonstop world we are constantly navigating. Whether you are overcoming an illness or navigating the day-to-day curveballs life throws at us, Seneca, an ancient Greek Stoic philosopher, warns us the greatest obstacle to living is expectancy. Live immediately and enjoy the process.

Seneca said, "True happiness is to enjoy the present, without anxious dependency upon the future, not to amuse ourselves with either hopes or fears but to rest satisfied with what we have."[69] We always think we are in control and no matter how hard we try, we are not. Trying to live in the moments of the day-to-day is such a fleeting concept to me. We constantly want more so quickly we forget to stop and appreciate the victories. If we do not learn to appreciate the little things in life and the daily process, then no matter what we do or accomplish, will ever be enough.

One of my favorite quotes from Paulo Coelho is when he described traveling, which epitomizes this very notion of living in the moment. He says, "When you travel, you experience, in a very practical way, the act of rebirth. You confront completely new situations, the day passes more slowly, and on most journeys, you don't even understand the language. So you are like a child out of the womb. You begin to attach much more importance to the things around you because your survival depends upon them. You begin to be more accessible to others because they might be able to help you in a difficulty situation. At the same time, since things are new, you see only the beauty in them, and you feel happy to be alive."[70]

So many of my patients tell me they wish they could appreciate the journey more versus the destination. We are so wired to do everything but live in the moment. We take in data from the present, compare with data from the past, then use that to make predictions about the future. This is constantly happening; it's so automatic we are perpetually living with this low level of anxiety. Traveling, trying new hobbies, art,

---

69   "Quotable Quote," Goodreads, accessed October 2, 2020.

70   Paulo Coelho, *The Pilgrimage* (San Francisco: Harper One, 2008), 35.

music, and overall experiences that violate our expectations based on this data processing is what life is all about. My patients have helped me understand this flow of the present and escaping the pattern of routine.

Living in the moment and being able to trust the process gets you one step closer to happiness in your recovery. Let's look at Jill Bolte Taylor's story. She was named one of *Time* magazine's "100 Most Influential People in the World" in 2008. Jill Bolte Taylor is a Harvard-trained brain scientist who suffered a massive stroke on the morning of December 10, 1996. In her book, *My Stroke of Insight*, she shares her unique perspective on the brain and its capacity for recovery. In one chapter, she discussed what she needed the most in her recovery that ultimately helped unlock her happiness. She starts by saying, "Recovery was a decision I had to make a million times a day."[71]

I found this very interesting. She had to choose over and over again to take part in the process of recovery. It did not simply take a single moment, but constant effort to establish a system that worked for her. The following three necessities she discusses also speak to the importance of focusing on the process and not the final product.

1. For a successful recovery, it was important to focus on her ability and not disability by celebrating achievements every day.

---

71   Jill Bolte Taylor, *My Stroke of Insight* (New York: The Penguin Group, 2006), 110.

2. She needed people to celebrate the triumphs she made every day because her successes, no matter how small, inspired her.

3. Her successful recovery was completely dependent on her ability to break every task down into smaller and simpler steps to action—not the end goal![72]

How can you shift your attention and energy from the final product to the process and does it really work?

The science supports the power of shifting our attention to the process as well. During my didactic work in physical therapy school, I loved learning about the anatomy and function of the brain. My favorite part is a system called the Reticular Activating System (RAS). It is essentially the attention center. It is the filter between subconscious and conscious mind. Ever notice when you go shopping for a car you love, you suddenly see that car everywhere? That is your RAS at work. The RAS seeks information that validates your beliefs and takes what we focus on and creates a filter for it. It will only allow through what is important to us.[73] In the rehabilitation realm, if you are able to focus your attention on the systems in place to get to your goal, your RAS will reveal the people, information, and opportunities that help you achieve them. This will allow you to see the good in the moment and live more immediately.

---

72   Taylor, *My Stroke of Insight*, 118.

73   "If You Want It, You Might Get It. The Reticular Activating System Explained," Desk of Van Schneider (blog), accessed April 3, 2020.

In James Clear's book, *Atomic Habits*, he has this notion of focusing on the systems in place versus the actual end goal, which resonated with me and how I discuss my patient's recovery from the start. He says, "Goals are about the results you want to achieve. Systems are about the processes that lead to those results."[74] While I believe setting goals is important, the second part of Clear's argument is the key. One example he uses is of any coach. Your goal will be to win a championship, but your system is how you recruit players, manage your assistant coaches, and run practices. You can't sit there and watch the score board every game just hoping the score will magically have you win.

Additionally, you cannot just say you want to get back to the way you were performing certain things without a system in place. Clear says a systems-first mentality provides the antidote. Like my patient, Maddi, Clear asserts, "When you fall in love with the process rather than the product, you don't have to wait to give yourself permission to be happy."[75] With my patients, there is more than one system that can get you to your final destination. Everyone has to find what works for them to set them on the road to recovery. Lastly, systems are meant to be changed and modified along the way. There is more than one path to success.

One of the most powerful messages Inky Johnson posted on his Instagram epitomizes this chapter's message and the narrative I paint with my patients: "Don't get stuck in the

---

74   James Clear, *Atomic Habits* (New York: Penguin Random House, 2018), 23.

75   Clear, *Atomic Habits*, 26.

past, and don't try to fast forward yourself into a future you haven't earned....Give today all the love, intensity, gratitude, and courage you can."[76] As long as your system is running, you can be happy at any time and enjoy the process.

76   Inky Johnson(@inkyjohnson), Instagram photo, August 17, 2020.

PART 3

LIVES TOUCHED AND LESSONS LEARNED

CHAPTER 9

INTOKU

———

*"One is only as happy in proportion
as he makes others feel happy."*

MILTON HERSHEY

Hindsight is twenty-twenty. I was listening to Ed Mylett's podcast and he said to his guest something that resonated with me on a very personal level. He articulated the adage of hindsight but in a more pragmatic way that helps with reflecting on points in my life.

He said, "Hindsight on our life is one of the greatest evidences of our faith."[77]

If we just look back and reflect, we can see there was a plan and preparation there for us. It is clear to me the way I grew up and my experiences helped guide me and gave me the

---

77 Ed Mylett, "Perspective Drives Performance with Inky Johnson," February 5, 2020, *The Ed Mylett Show*, podcast, MP3 audio, 27:00.

tools to excel in my career. In life, we model behaviors of our heroes and people who made a difference in our lives. As I reflected on the lessons I learned from patients in my career, I now appreciate much more the human connection and empathy my dad demonstrated on a daily basis in his career. I wanted to understand, not so much the actions, but the spirit that drove his acts treating the customers and the people he served for twenty-five years in an inner city setting.

My parents emigrated from Jordan in the late 1970s in the pursuit of Thomas Jefferson's fundamental right of the pursuit of happiness. Around the time Italy was beating Germany in the 1982 World Cup and Michael Jackson's *Thriller* album was released, my parents were purchasing a liquor store business in Jersey City, New Jersey. The store was located in the Greenville section of Jersey City. It is the Southernmost section of the urban city. This inner city neighborhood is predominantly African-American in population and to say my dad stood out was an understatement.

Like a lot of the neighborhoods around Jersey City, Greenville's brick row houses are prevalent. Ocean One Stop, the name of my dad's store, was nestled on the bottom of a three-story brick building with two residential apartments on top. The entrance to the narrow liquor store housed a vestibule where customers would have to speak through a bulletproof glass window to place an order. My dad would get the requested item from the shelves behind him, ring up the customer, and place the item in a drawer before pushing the drawer closed for the customer to grab. That was the reality of the environment he was in. He lived in this reality for nearly twenty-five years.

Although the dangers were ever present, I never really thought my dad worked in a treacherous environment. He never let me work with him like he did my older brother because of the threatening atmosphere. My dad was in the store twelve to fifteen hours a day. Through it all, he provided a sense of stability for his customers who adored him in a relatively turbulent urban city. He would provide jobs for certain people of the area to keep them off the streets and out of trouble. The customers protected my dad in the event he ever ran into any trouble—a testament to the human connection my dad had with those he served.

My fondest memory as I reflected on my dad's time in the store was how we would spend our Thanksgiving. I would be lying if I were able to appreciate and grasp the magnitude of my parents' actions every year on our annual tradition. As most of my friends and their families were getting ready to spend their Thanksgiving dinners at home, we would help my mom prep the necessities to bring with us to the store to have our Thanksgiving dinner with my dad. Not only did my mom prepare a turkey for my family, but also cooked another two turkeys to feed the customers and local community.

This particular holiday has its own array of aromas that have ingrained themselves into my memories of family and friends. Our thirty-minute drive from home to the store and the anticipation that came with it is one of my oldest and most cherished memories. I remember the lines would form, the laughter shared, and the countless stories told as we sat in the safety of the narrow liquor store on various cases of liquor. Watching my dad interact with such authenticity and empathy for his customers, I now know, laid the foundation for my career path and instilled in me one of my greatest strengths: empathy and the power to connect and feel deeply. I feel emotions for others and I can see it—the pure happiness and joy people experience. Conversely, I also feel raw and real sadness. At times, it consumes me. As I practice reflection in my life, I am now able to better manage and proactively use my empathy to help my patients.

Reflection, I am learning, is more than looking back and just thinking about moments that made us happy or sad. I am learning to appreciate and transform these experiences into genuine learning and growth to apply them moving forward. I have learned over the past few years just how powerful this practice of reflection can be. My patients have taught me so much and the rest of this chapter dives into the first of the three lessons they have taught me. These lessons have helped me begin to unlock the happiness perspective in my own life and it can help you do the same.

~ ~ ~

"INTOKU"

The warm feeling you get when you have done something for someone else is not just in your head. It is, in fact, chemicals in your brain responding to these acts of kindness. These simple acts have the potential to release hormones that help your mood and overall well-being and is even being used in psychotherapy as a treatment for certain diagnoses, such as depression. The primary chemical released is oxytocin. Dr. Waguih William Ishak is a professor of psychiatry at Cedars-Sinai, a nonprofit hospital in Los Angeles. He reports studies link random acts of kindness to releasing dopamine in the brain that is responsible for giving us a feeling of happiness. Additionally, helping others is also believed to increase levels of Substance P, which helps with pain modulation in our bodies. Dr. Ishak says, "Small acts of kindness help us feel better and they help those who receive them. We are building better selves and better communities at the same time."[78] *The first lesson my patients have taught me is how the smallest acts of kindness can have the biggest impact in people's lives.*

The majority of patients I treat will typically spend a prolonged period of time away from home and in a hospital setting. During that time, or even when they return home, they often tell me how visits from family and friends or simple texts or phone calls helped them during their recovery process. Maddi attributes part of her recovery to the small acts of kindness she received during her recovery. She said, "The prayers and positive thoughts from those I knew and loved as well as strangers completely changed the trajectory of my recovery."[79] It does not have to be a grandiose, elaborate act to have a lasting impact on someone. My patients are constantly reminding me the little things, prayer cards, home-cooked dinners, gifts, and letters often have the most impact. Whether it is in the recovery realm or in the day-to-day journey of life, coming from a place of collaboration rather than competition allows us move humanity forward, one small act of kindness at a time.

---

78   "The Science of Kindness," Cedars-Sinai, accessed April 17, 2020.

79   Madeline Niebanck, conversation with author, March 26, 2020.

Consider the personal account of my parent's accident I mentioned earlier and how a small act of kindness made all the difference for my family. December 27, 2017 will be a day I will never forget and has forever changed my perspective on answering unknown phone numbers. My brother and I were sitting on my couch watching Villanova basketball take care of the Blue Demons from DePaul University when his phone rang. After two or three rings, I looked over at him and he said, "I never answer unknown numbers." I turned my attention back to the TV and, after another ring, he answered the phone with a routine "hello." If I am being honest, the next three to four hours were a blur, but I will try to recount what I can. My brother stood up from the couch and his voice changed to panic as he said, "What do you mean my parents were in a bad car accident?"

My parents had left my apartment about thirty minutes earlier. Without thinking, I called my neighbor, a cop in town, and explained as calmly as I could the call we just received while at the same time hearing my brother yelling into the phone—it was chaos. I heard all of this while trying to get my shoes and socks on and got into my car thinking the absolute worst.

We found out where they took my parents after numerous phone calls. My neighbor called us back on our ride down and said the car was completely totaled. He could see my dad was doing okay, but he wasn't too sure about my mom amidst all the police lights and ambulances. Because of the setting I work in and knowing all the possible injuries that could have happened, they started to scan through my head on our ride to the emergency room: brain injury, spinal cord injury resulting in paralysis, weakness, aphasia, gait impairments, bracing, assistive device use, durable medical equipment, G-tube, Foley catheter, Hoyer lift, stair lift, commodes, field cuts, so on and so forth. Sometimes I wish I did not work in this setting and know what I know—there really is something to be said of the notion "ignorance is bliss."

My brother and I arrived at the hospital and realized while my dad had a few bumps and bruises, he was okay. My parents both had their seat belts on and God knows what could have been otherwise. When we saw my mom, she was lying on her side in what appeared to be the worst pain imaginable. There was something extremely humbling about seeing both my parents on stretchers. I see patients every single day in wheelchairs and stretchers when they come with a transportation service to receive therapy with me, but this was a sight I had never experienced. My mom was diagnosed with a fractured posterior wall of her acetabulum and a dislocated hip, which ultimately needed surgical intervention; however, before they could do anything, they needed to reduce (put her hip back in place) or it could lead to compromised blood flow to the area and more complications. To put things in perspective, my brother, a vascular surgeon, who sees gunshot wounds, stabbings, and severe trauma cases, had to walk away from my mom's screaming and yelling when they reduced her hip back in place.

Knowing where to go in the event of medical issues is just as important in the potential for healing as the injury itself. I highly recommend doing research and knowing which hospitals are in your area and what exactly they are equipped for. Being proactive is so much better than being reactive when it comes to health care. Ignorance can be bliss, but knowledge is power and when we found out the extent of the surgery and injury, I was overcome by an extreme sense of calm knowing about the outcomes of this particular procedure.

After surgery, my mom was non-weight bearing for eight weeks. She also had hip precautions, which was another obstacle. She could not move her hip in certain positions or else it could dislocate. My brother looked after her during the day and I would arrive after work and do more therapy with her. Seeing my brother in the room while I was doing some exercises was quite comical. He would ask me questions like, "Are you sure she can move like that? Are you sure she can do that exercise?" I would often say to him to leave the room or go do a surgery. She also needed to learn non-weight bearing status for walking with the rolling walker by hopping. She progressed extremely well and after my brother took care of the surgery and hospital stay, it was time to transfer my mom to my acute rehabilitation hospital.

I have spent the past eight years in this hospital and for some reason, I foolishly thought a family member would never be a patient. Seeing people every day in a very vulnerable state is humbling and I try to treat my patients as if they are a member of my own family. I would be lying if I said it was easy to do that day in and day out, but I certainly try. Walking in and out of work over the years, I saw patients' family members arriving or leaving to visit their loved ones. I would finish work and go up to my mom's room to see how her day was. Leaving and arriving to work has a different feeling for me now; that experience helped me to appreciate all the support, visits, and well wishes we received and how integral it was to have that support system. Being vulnerable as a patient and as family members is not easy and it gave me a new perspective on helping and supporting others.

My mom was finally discharged January 13, 2018 and the house was all set for her arrival. My mom was still not allowed to put any weight on her leg, so the stairs to her bedroom were out of the question. The hospital bed was set up on the first floor and would be her new bedroom for the next six weeks. My sister, who lived in Dubai at the time, probably took this the hardest since she was so far away. The flights for her to come home with such short notice were astronomically priced, and a coworker of hers, along with her husband, gifted my sister a round-trip flight home using their miles. I still think of this act of kindness and smile from time to time. We surprised my parents and their reaction when my sister arrived left me forever indebted to that act of kindness that has had such a lasting impact on my family.

I am a stout believer of things happening for a reason. God has a plan and puts us through experiences and situations to make us stronger. I learned a great deal during this experience and am so thankful my parents had their seat belts on, because I know how much worse this could have been. Personally, I feel this strengthened my relationship with my parents, as well as gave them a better understanding of what I do in my profession.

Lastly, it helped me recharge my batteries and appreciate how important it is to continue to try to treat every single one of my patients as family members, because the vulnerable state they are in is challenging beyond words. The triumph of the human spirit is something I am in awe of every day. We joke all the time that my dad would not be able to handle what my mom went through. The strength my mom had during the whole process is a microcosm of the strength she has shown my siblings and I my whole life. Something I try to emulate in my daily mindset.

On Instagram, I follow the 2017 iPhone app of the year called *Calm*. Random phrases or quotes pop up when I open Instagram from time to time and one that popped up and sticks with me is "Intoku," from a Japanese proverb that means "good done in secret, specifically the act of doing good secretly, for its own sake."[80] Small acts of kindness can have the biggest therapeutic effect on those around us. Be sincere in your kindness and honesty so you will not only help others, but yourself as well.

---

80   Alan Newton, "Practicing Intoku," *Executive Summary Magazine*, November 25, 2017.

CHAPTER 10

THE POWER OF HUMAN CONNECTION

———

"There isn't time, so brief is life, for bickerings, apologies, heartburnings, callings to account. There is only time of loving and but an instant, so to speak, for that. The good life is built with good relationships."

MARK TWAIN

In an interview with Oprah Winfrey, Queen Rania of Jordan said, "Once you feel that others are like you, then you want for others what you want for yourself."[81] She was explaining how one of her biggest goals in raising her children is to make sure they feel connected to the world. She wants them to be global citizens. Human connection is something we all want.

———

81   Queen Rania, "Queen Rania Speaks with Oprah on Oprah Show," May 17, 2006, video, 1:20.

Connecting with my patients is something I pride myself on and I have leaned into over the past few years. When I have a strong connection with my patients, it deepens the moment, inspires change, and builds trust.

One thing my patients have taught me is to better understand these connections. I go to work every single day and have numerous opportunities to connect with others. My patients put their trust in me with their rehabilitation process. During my interactions with them, I cultivate strong bonds and learn about the power of connecting with others and the impact it can have. *The second lesson my patients have taught me is the power of human connection.* I learned just how impactful connecting with others can be from a late patient of mine.

"Code Blue outpatient parking lot. Code Blue outpatient parking lot. Code Blue outpatient parking lot."

Those words always freeze me in my tracks when I am at work. Code Blue indicates a medical emergency. November 23, 2018, Black Friday, took on a brand new meaning for me as well as my patient and his family. My patient, who I will refer to as DD, was enjoying his Thanksgiving dinner with his wife and family twelve hours earlier. Prior to this particular code being called, I had completed my hour-long session with him in an Ekso-skeleton device. Ekso Bionics is a company that develops and manufactures powered Ekso-skeleton devices strapped on as wearable robots to enhance the strength, mobility, and endurance of soldiers' paraplegics. These robots have a variety of applications in the medical, military, industrial, and consumer markets. It enables individuals with any amount of lower extremity weakness, including those who are paralyzed, to stand up and walk.

In July of 2005, my patient had a rapid onset of weakness, numbness, and functional decline. He had a condition known as a spinal arterio-venous malformation: a very rare abnormal tangle of blood vessels that disrupts the blood flow to the surrounding cells, depriving them of vital oxygen and causing cells in spinal tissue to deteriorate or die. The area in the spinal cord in which this occurs dictates the severity of impairments in the patients. My patient had suffered the spinal cord injury at the mid-thoracic level, leaving him essentially paralyzed from the waist down and relying on his wheelchair as a primary means of mobility.

I had known my patient for a few years by the time we started using the Ekso robot during this round of therapy. I had seen him multiple times in traditional therapy, and over the course of my time with him, we developed a very strong bond and shared a lot of the same interests; Big East basketball being at the top of the list. He was an avid Seton Hall Pirates fan so college basketball season was always a great time for both of us. My patient's son studied abroad in Newcastle, so the English premiere league was a frequent point of discussion during our seven o'clock physical therapy sessions. I always knew we had a strong bond, but it would not be until this Code Blue occurred I realized just how impactful simple conversations and connections could actually be.

After walking about five hundred feet in the robot and sitting back down in his wheelchair, my patient had a follow up appointment with his doctor. About twenty minutes later, he returned to the gym to get his jacket. We exchanged a few laughs and discussed the premier league match-ups that weekend for my Arsenal squad taking on Bournemouth and his Newcastle team matched up against Burnley. All of a sudden, Code Blue was announced and my heart rate immediately started to climb. I jogged out of the waiting area and toward the outpatient exit. Once I got outside, I immediately felt the cold winter air pierce through my sweater and deep into my bones.

A man was walking toward me and yelled, "The car back there is moving backwards in reverse, just going in circles!"

As I picked up my pace toward the car, I noticed exactly who it was and went into a dead sprint. Being the first one on the scene, the timing of my arrival and the way the driver side door aligned with me was nothing short of miraculous. My patient, who just wished me a great weekend a few minutes ago, was now unresponsive with his seatbelt fastened and going in reverse about ten miles per hour in circles. I sprung open the unlocked door—again, a miracle—and pressed the brake with my left hand and with my right hand put the car in park.

I ripped the seat belt off, yelling his name as he struggled to breathe. My colleague helped get him out of the car and I was unable to get a pulse. She started CPR and 9-1-1 was called. Our code team arrived, including doctors and nurses, and he was connected to a monitor with no pulse. Bagging was initiated to help with breathing and an IV was inserted into his arm. Within about two minutes (which felt like an hour), the patient had some spontaneous breathing and a very faint pulse. Vitals were monitored as CPR continued until the paramedics came and took him to the local hospital. He passed away five days later.

His wife, whom I had never met before and only heard about through my interactions with him, called me at work and left me the following message, which shook me to my core.

"Farris, this is DD's wife. I am sorry to tell you this, but DD passed this morning. I can't begin to tell you how he felt about you. All he talked about was Farris and how much you helped him, and if I can use the word LOVE, he really LOVED you. I am sorry to bring you this news, but even trying to revive him on Friday was beyond any angel; but thank you and I am sorry to pass this sad news."[82]

A woman I have never met before just lost her husband and took the time to call me and let me know on that same day. The connection I had with her husband was way beyond anything I could have ever imagined. He taught me our interactions with those who cross our path is an opportunity to spread love. You never know the effect our interactions can have on those around us and it does not cost anything to spread kindness. Another reflection point from my relationship with this patient was his ability to help me realize and shape my self-worth (which is transient). With social media being what it is today, society is constantly looking outward for self-worth and reassurance in a variety of different areas of our lives.

---

82   Voice message to author, November 30, 2018.

One area my self-worth comes from is my real connections with people. I pride myself and judge myself based on how many people are good to me, help me, and how many people I can help. I want to dive into the power of human connection a bit more to understand how we can get better. It is a skill and with practice, we can improve.

As I continued to conduct interviews and performed more research on the power and importance of human connection, I came across an episode from *The School of Greatness* podcast hosted by Lewis Howes. On this particular episode, he was interviewing Brian Grazer. Brian is an American film and television producer and cofounded Imagine Entertainment in 1986. Films he has produced have grossed over thirteen billion dollars. Some of the most notable movies and four for which Grazer was personally nominated for an Academy Award include *Splash*, *Apollo 13*, *A Beautiful Mind*, and *Frost/Nixon*. He won the Oscar for Best Picture for *A Beautiful Mind* and, in 2007, was named one of *Time*'s "100 Most Influential People in the World."

In the podcast, he discusses his book, *Face to Face: Stories on the Power of Human Connection*. While it might seem like second nature, Grazer proves eye contact is one of the most transformative habits you can develop in your daily life. Eye contact has the power to offer validation, show generosity, create intimacy, and most importantly, establish genuine human connection. Even as technology takes on a bigger and bigger role in our lives, from self-driving cars to the smartphones in our pockets, no machine will ever be able to replace the unique and powerful benefits of eye contact.

The catalyst for wanting to write his book was to share and reveal a secret to forge a happier and more successful life. It provides techniques to succeed and the importance of connecting with people. The narrative he paints really is the idea of human connection. To connect with people, you have to connect to their hearts. He says, "You have to look at people. You can't be looking at your phone or splitting your attention at all. People have to feel your sincerity, feel your heart, and be captivated by you in a real way."[83] Later in the interview, he describes the importance of eye contact; the way he explained it was perfect for the digital age we live in. He says, "Face to face, eyeball to eyeball connection is the Wi-Fi to human connection." Once you are on this connection, you can communicate with each other and begin to build a bond and trusting relationship.[84]

Early in my career this is something I struggled with. My first visit with any new patient is an initial evaluation. This entails me asking questions about their history of whatever injury they had. I will ask about their past medical history and their prior level of functioning and get as many pieces of the puzzle to try and paint a picture of how the patient was before their injury. This allows me to have insight and begin to formulate a plan of attack regarding what exercises would be appropriate for that particular patient. After going through the history and feeling comfortable with an understanding of what happened to my patient, I begin the objective portion of the evaluation where I check how

83   Lewis Howes, "The Art of Human Connection," October 29, 2019, in *The School of Greatness* podcast, video, 24:25.

84   Ibid.

they are currently able to move and function. I will check things like their strength, range of motion in their joints, their ability to transfer from a chair to a standing position, their balance, and if they can perform these tasks, walking and stairs. Once I get through my evaluation, I explain my findings and let them know my game plan and make sure we are on the same page.

My first few years as a physical therapist, I thought the objective testing to see how they were able to perform certain activities was the most important; so much so I found myself often thinking about what test I was going to perform with them instead of listening to their response to a question I just asked. I have come to appreciate and learn, from the moment I first introduce myself to a new patient until the moment I wrap up my evaluation with them, I have to cultivate a connection or else it will impact their rehabilitation. Now, there are times when I take the entire evaluation and just talk to my patients to build a strong foundation and never get to any testing until my second visit. By building a strong rapport with my patients in that regard, I have seen them engaged much more in the rehabilitation process. I notice they do not miss as many visits and are more compliant with their home exercise program as I begin to give them exercises to perform at home and empower them along the way.

Dan Scwabel, *New York Times* bestselling author, states in his book, *Back to Human*, just how powerful human connection is. His book relates to the workforce and how that connection creates greater fulfillment and productivity. He created the work connectivity index tool that measures the strength of one's relationships at work. Dan dedicated his work to studying how the connections we make in the workspace can impact productivity and overall well-being.

Online and mobile technologies have created the illusion that today's workers feel highly connected to one another, but in reality, most feel isolated. He highlights how technology has made us on call twenty-four hours per day and seven days per week. On the podcast, he argues technology has created an illusion of connection. He reports "we touch our cell phones every fifteen minutes and twenty-six hundred times a day!"[85] We have to use technology properly. He asserts we should be using technology to get people to a specific place, but once we are there, we should be physically present and listen to people and others around us to cultivate relationships and lasting connections. In a study consisting of two thousand people globally, he found that 10 percent of people have zero friends at work and half of the work force have fewer than five friends at work.[86]

In January of 2020, Cigna released their 2020 Loneliness Report; it was mind-boggling to me. They reported 61 percent of Americans are lonely, which is up from 54 percent in 2018.[87] Additionally, this percentage equates to over 201 million people. They found people are lonely because of a lack of meaningful interactions and social support. It amazes me how we have every opportunity to connect with others

85   Lewis Howes, "Building Human Connection in a Digital World," November 11, 2018, in *The School of Greatness* podcast, video, 7:40.

86   Lewis Howes, "Building Human Connection in a Digital World," November 11, 2018, in *The School of Greatness* podcast, video, 5:20.

87   Dan Schawbel (@danschawbel), Instagram photo, January 21, 2020.

through different social media and technological advances yet lack the human connection in so many different areas of our lives. Whether we look at human connection in our personal lives or in the working sector, the need to establish relationships and connecting with others is imperative. My patients have taught me the importance of working on this habit. It is indeed a skill we can work on and something I continuously strive to improve upon.

So how can we combat loneliness we are facing and improve our human connection? The science supports positive impacts it can have and we are just scratching the surface of how bad this pandemic of loneliness really is. Did you know the ATM we all use stands for "automated teller machine"? I did not. Donald Wetzel came up with the idea of the ATM in 1968 and the rest, as they say, is history. He was waiting in line and the idea occurred to him during a twenty-minute wait to see the teller in the bank. In her *Happiness Lab* podcast, Dr. Laurie Santos discusses the cost of saving time and avoiding these bank lines and other lines—a social cost. Lines give us an opportunity to be around other people. She interviewed Don and his wife about the ATM. Interestingly, Donald's wife, Eleanor, has never used an ATM. She always uses a bank teller. Eleanor says, "The ATM does not smile back at you."[88]

Consider technology and a routine daily practice most of us partake in every single morning: getting coffee. Starbucks and other companies now offer orders through their

---

88   Dr. Laurie Santos, "Mistakenly Seeking Solitude," October 8, 2019, in *The Happiness Lab*, produced by Pushkin, podcast, MP3 audio, 14:40.

application on the phone so you can place an order in the comfort of your car or home, go right into the store, grab your coffee, not say a word to anyone, and be on your way. No conversation, human interaction, or connection at all. You may think this is more efficient as you read this; what a great invention! However, it is exacerbating the problem of feeling alone and unhappy.

In 2015, I was having a conversation with a friend. At the time he had just moved here from Italy and we were talking about the differences between our cultures. I asked him what he missed the most and his response was not one I was expecting; quite frankly, I didn't fully understand at the time. He paused for a second and said, "The moment of the coffee." The few minutes when you are having a cafe with someone, sharing those few minutes to discuss and *connect* is something I can truly appreciate now.

Perhaps you can try ordering your coffee with the barista next time you seek out your caffeine fix. This constant practice can have lasting effects on your overall health and well-being. Give it a shot (of espresso) if you like!

CHAPTER 11

AIM HIGHER

———

"Normal is overrated. Aim higher."

BONNIE ST. JOHN

The definition of normal is conforming to a type, standard, or regular pattern. It comes from a Latin word *normalis*, which described something made with a carpenter's square. Something built this way would be normed to have angles perfectly aligned and fit a general pattern. It was adopted into English in the seventeenth century. Normal is defined as "conforming to a type, standard, or regular pattern: characterized by that which is considered usual, typical, or routine."[89] It has taken me some time to appreciate this, but I never use the word normal when it comes to my patients' recovery. I try to redirect them and shift the narrative from a normal way to a new way to achieve their goals.

———

89   *Merriam-Webster*, s.v. "normal (adj.)," accessed September 29, 2020.

My patients consistently ask questions like the ones listed below:

"Am I ever going to walk normally?"

"Is my leg ever going to move normally?"

"Am I ever going to be normal again?"

The third lesson my patients have taught me is to reframe in my own life and in how I treat my patients what the notion of normal really means. There is a sense of built-in biases when one uses the word "normal." During my didactic work in physical therapy school, I learned how the body worked and operated, and specifically how it related to function. One of the functional tasks I look at every single day is someone's gait, or how they walk. In school we would learn the "normal" way to walk, looking at things like weight shifting, foot clearance, step length and width, and posture. As I reflected on this, I realized there is no normal way of walking. The way I walk and the way you walk are not normal by any means. They are unique to our body types, experiences, and history.

I always find it interesting when a patient asks me if they will ever be able to walk "normally" after they have had a stroke or brain injury. None of my patients will ever be normal or get back to 100 percent. No matter how much progress my patients make, I never strive for them to be "normal." My goal is for them to become better from where they currently are. Every day I try to help them achieve their goals. I believe normal is a fluid sort of thing and when someone believes they are not doing something normally, it elicits a negative connotation which usually sets my patients up for failure. Normal is subjective and our societal constructs have led us to believe otherwise.

The reality is we are, of course, human, and more often than I would like, we get frustrated when we revert back to comparing our abilities to some sort of "normal" standard. Early in the rehabilitation process, this notion of normal distracts my patients from the more important task at hand or what they could do next to improve in the moment. The lens through which most of my patients view their recovery early on is one that distorts their ability to see the present. Often their conscious state is anchored much to the way they were prior to their injuries.

I went to a lecture given by Bonnie St. John at Seton Hall University. Bonnie is a former Olympic skier, author, and public speaker. Bonnie had her right leg amputated above the knee when she was five years old. Despite these challenges, she went on to excel as an athlete, scholar, and businesswoman. St. John is the first African-American to win medals in Winter Paralympic competitions as a ski racer and the first African-American to receive a medal in any Paralympic event, earning bronze and silver medals in several alpine skiing events during the 1984 Winter Paralympics. After graduating from Harvard and earning a Rhodes scholarship, St. John went on to have a successful corporate career, first in sales with IBM, then as a corporate consultant. She has written six books and at this particular lecture, she discussed the notion of micro-resilience specifically with her rehabilitation process and learning how to use her prosthesis.

She recounts one of her memories early in her rehabilitation process. Having her leg amputated at such an early age required countless visits to Shriners Hospital in Los Angeles. During her lecture, she described how, when she would go back to the hospital, it was a form of time travel for her. As we boarded her time travel machine, I was captivated by her story of perseverance and grit. She recounted nights of screaming in her sleep, surgeries for her leg, and hours of crying in physical therapy. Being able to go back to that hospital over the past few years to give back is something she is very passionate about. She now enjoys going there and meeting the current patients. She recognizes the impact of giving back and the impact it has on countless children just beginning their own fights.

Bonnie discussed the end of a visit at Shriners. She met a mother who was seated in the back of the large room she was in. The mother had her arm around her thirteen-year-old son who was badly burned on his face and arms.

The mother asked Bonnie, "Do you think my son will ever lead a normal life?"

Bonnie paused for a moment and replied, "I hope not. He should aim higher!"[90]

Through her experiences, Bonnie learned every single one of us can be extraordinary and unique. Normal is overrated. What society calls "normal" often times has an underlying tone of "perfection."

---

90   Bonnie St. John, Lecture, October 11, 2018 at Seton Hall University.

This response resonated with me. Something my patients have taught me, in line with Bronnie, is learned regret of living a life true to oneself. My patients are always so quick to compare their rehabilitation and progress with other patients in the gym. Teddy Roosevelt once said "comparison is the thief of joy." Everyone is different and has their own struggles and battles they are facing. There is no "normal." We have to be true to who we are and only compare ourselves to our own expectations and where we see ourselves, not to where others see us at the end of the day. Be happy with the effort you put forth, knowing you gave it your all and be happy with the outcome no matter what others say.

We should always aim higher. Aim higher and never settle until you are doing your best at any given time. Aim higher toward what moves you and what you are passionate about, not what others tell you to do or be. The most important key here is "aiming higher" and the height to which you should be reaching should be set by no one else but YOU! Your parents, your friends, physical therapists, or family shouldn't choose for you.

To me, aiming higher means focusing on trying to get better every single day. Let's rewind the clock to 2008 during my time at Villanova University. As I mentioned earlier, I was a member of the men's soccer team and during my senior year, I was fortunate enough to be named co-captain with my good friend, Joey Taylor. We would meet with our head coach, Tom Carlin, regularly and he introduced us to a Japanese term: kaizen. It was our mantra for the season and has taken me some time and reflection to truly grasp the meaning of the word.

Kaizen means "change for the better" or "continuous improvement." My coach was trying to build a culture where we were focusing on the process of trying to get better every single day, practice, game, or meeting. We were not focusing on winning games or the final product. If we can just focus on what we need to do to get better, that is all we can control. Aiming higher, in recovery and life in general, means focusing on what we can control and trying to become a better version of ourselves day by day. This is a lesson my coach instilled in me and my patients have reinforced. A lesson I am confident has helped me begin to unlock my happiness and pray it does the same for you.

In an earlier chapter, I mentioned the idea of reference points and their impact on happiness. Like other realms of our lives, my patients tend to pick reference points that rob them of happiness during their recovery. Being "normal" as a reference point sets us up for failure. Frankly, our minds are terrible at picking standards to compare. I see this to be even more prevalent and challenging with my patients after trauma. I do recognize a reference point during recovery and trauma lends itself to picking someone's old "normal" self as the standard. For example: "I can walk with a cane now but I cannot walk like I used to prior to my stroke; I can go up ten steps now but I have to go one step at a time versus being able to go up normally." My patients have taught me to reframe how I look at the word "normal" and understand aiming higher means picking the right reference point to guide my happiness compass.

Dr. Laurie Santos discusses different strategies to break out of our minds annoying feature of adaptation. A powerful strategy that helps my patients and myself break the mindset of looking at normal as the gold standard is the idea of *negative visualization*. If you are able to intentionally practice this habit, we can get out of the mindset of playing the victim or not being able to get back to "normal." By doing this, we reframe our mindset to focus on how the injury could have been a little worse. "What if my stroke was in a different part of my brain where I was not able to walk at all?" Having this moment and thought process can help in getting us out of the habit of looking at our old self and appreciate what can be done currently.[91]

Thinking about losing the ability to move your leg, walk with a walker, or go up a few steps can help reframe one's perspective and how one looks at "normal." When you do this and the dust settles, you can see "normal" is now no longer relevant, because the good things come to the forefront. You are now seeing the ability to walk with a walker, going up the stairs one step at a time, or your ability to transfer from your wheelchair to the bed independently as things that might be lost and you are now appreciative and thankful for the ability to perform such tasks.

In my interview with Eric LeGrand, he defined happiness as "waking up every day, knowing that you have an opportunity to attack that day. To make the best of that day. Another opportunity to go out there and change someone else's life while changing your life at the same time." He went on to give me his definition of success that ties in perfectly with

---

91   Laurie Santos, "The Science of Well-Being," Yale University, Part One—Thwart Hedonic Adaptation, video, 7:45.

what aiming higher means. He defines success as "the peace of mind you get knowing you did everything you could to be the best you can be."[92] Aiming higher is not about trying to be normal, but it is about trying to improve and become a better version of yourself on a daily basis.

My patients have taught me to aim higher in my personal and professional endeavors and stay true to what makes me happy. In doing so, I can minimize any regrets moving forward. This lesson is something I carry with me in my daily mindset and I'm thankful I have been able to reflect and recognize. Having this new perspective has helped me unlock my own happiness over the past few years. No one knows what the future holds, but day in and day out, we get to choose to constantly aim higher. Life is not perfect or easy and I am now able to appreciate that the word "normal" houses certain biases that set us up for failure. When you give it your all and follow what you are passionate about, you can live with the results. There is always work to be done and room for improvement, and aiming higher is the way to keep moving forward.

---

92   Eric LeGrand, conversation with author, March 27, 2020.

CHAPTER 12

CONCLUSION

"Most folks are as happy as they
make up their minds to be."

ABRAHAM LINCOLN

I love to travel, and one of my favorite places I have been is the Dead Sea in Jordan. This is where my parents emigrated from. There is a plethora of history there and it is truly one of the most unique places I have had the opportunity to experience. Dead is defined as "deprived of life...lacking power to move, feel, or respond."[93] I felt the complete opposite when I was at the Dead Sea. As I worked my way down the various flights of stairs through the Arab village-like resort to the water, I could see the amazing panorama of the entire length of the sea. Prior to the narrow wooden walkway leading to the water, I massaged the Dead Sea mud all over my body. Once it dried, I was ready. The water was a gorgeous jade and I plotted the best strategy to avoid

---

93   *Merriam-Webster*, s.v. "dead *(adj.)*," accessed March 2, 2020.

the rocks upon entrance into the silky filmed water. After deciding, I plunged myself into the water and immediately surrendered to the incredible buoyancy of the water. It felt like I was wearing a life vest and it is the most indescribable feeling I have experienced.

For a place known for having no life, I could not be more alive both physically and emotionally. My senses firing and floating in the Dead Sea at sunset was truly a magical experience I will never forget. When viewed from the wrong lens, death is a finite state of being overwhelmed with negative connotations. If the Dead Sea can provide so many vibrant and lively emotions and be such a place of serenity, maybe looking at death, obstacles, and trauma in this perspective can help you live your life with a little more buoyancy—unlocking your own happiness along the way.

~ ~ ~

This book uniquely combines keys to unlocking one's happiness as it relates to physical trauma and the science behind those keys. I wanted to write this book because I feel so strongly that unlocking one's happiness depends tremendously on the lens in which one looks at their life. I want to close with a few final thoughts. The four keys to unlocking your happiness are based on my experiences with my patients. You can grow into each one and I want you to be patient and kind. Appreciate the small gains along the way and take the time to appreciate the little victories, because if you do not, nothing you accomplish or achieve in this marathon of life will ever be enough.

Throughout the book, we've looked at stories about overcoming life-changing injuries. We've met patients with spinal cord injuries, strokes, and amputations. Each of these people have faced different circumstances, but ultimately unlocked their happiness in the same way: through altruism, gratitude, trusting the process, and not letting moments of doubt turn into a mindset of surrender. Unfortunately, there is no thermometer to measure happiness. Happiness is very subjective; what makes one person happy does not necessarily make the next person happy. It is transient and something that ebbs and flows. Not every day is going to be perfect. You will have good days and bad days.

When it comes to happiness as it relates to physical trauma or any other area of your life, I recognize there are constant choices that need to be made. There are days and situations where giving up is the best action to take. As I highlighted early, it is okay to have those days. Lean into them when they manifest, but know YOU WILL come out stronger. We need to constantly exercise our happiness muscle. The more we exercise and flex our happiness muscle, the more satisfied we will be with the efforts we put in.

Happiness is indeed a choice. I wholeheartedly agree with this notion, but with my experiences, it is so much more than a single choice. Another way to think about happiness is a culmination of choices one makes on a daily basis. Indecision is a choice. When you do not make a decision about an obstacle, you are in a constant state of weighing options, which is no longer living in the present. Make a decision even if it is a wrong decision for a particular situation. You can at least learn from it and make the right decision moving forward.

Happiness is a process that takes daily discipline and practice. It is not an end goal. Unlocking your happiness means waking up every morning trying to be better than yesterday's version of oneself. It means constantly moving forward, whether that means stepping, rolling, or pushing, even when you do not think you can. If you are unable to do something on your first attempt, DO NOT give up. You need to try again or try a different way. Ask for help because people are willing to help. "Good relationships don't just protect our bodies; they protect our brains,"[94] said Waldinger in his TED Talk. Surround yourself with people who will continuously build you up so on days you feel like stopping, you'll get a little push to keep moving forward.

This was a perfect time to launch a book about setbacks and overcoming obstacles. COVID-19 has come along as a major setback for the entire world. People, now more than ever, are questioning the philosophy of life. I mentioned Seneca in an earlier chapter; he was a Stoic. Stoicism was developed two thousand years ago by other philosophers like Marcus Aurelius, Epictetus, and Seneca. Stoics were all about minimizing negative emotions. William Irvine is a philosophy professor at Wright State University and the author of *The Stoic Challenge*. In his book, he discusses how some people bounce back in response to setbacks and others break. Stoics discovered that thinking of obstacles and challenges as tests of character can dramatically alter how

---

94   Robert Waldinger, "What Makes a Good Life? Lessons from the Longest Study on Happiness." November 2015, TED video, 8:54.

we respond to them.[95] I love the fundamental principles of Stoicism and believe we are in our own Stoic Renaissance of trying to understand life amidst all of our current obstacles and setbacks. We have to accept there are things we cannot control. We can achieve happiness, but it takes work. There is no quick fix to get happier, but the science shows there *is* a fix.

~ ~ ~

To my fellow medical professionals near and far:

Every single day we have the opportunity to impact people's lives. DO NOT take this for granted. One of the best things about our jobs is we get to not only meet people from all walks of life, but do what we can to help them. Sometimes we never get a chance to tell people how much they mean to us and what a difference they've made. I am so grateful for this opportunity and the chance I have at this moment to thank you. I know some days can be exhausting and frustrating, but just understand our patients are grateful for all the small things we do for them. We get to help others get through trying times and "carry their cross" in their recovery.

Each and every one of us was put here to help others. Please remember whenever you are not feeling so good about your day, yourself, or a situation, it will pass if you let it. Today is another day we have to impact others and make more memories moving humanity forward. Adele Levine, the author

95   William B. Irvine, *The Stoic Challenge* (New York: W. W. Norton & Company, Inc., 2019).

of *Run, Don't Walk*, describes our job best stating we are in the front lines battling together in the trenches of humanity. Day in and day out, you help people you've never met or may never meet again. It is more than just our occupation—it is our higher calling. Embrace and lean into this honor. You are exactly where you need to be.

ACKNOWLEDGMENTS

This journey has been everything I could have ever imagined and more. I never thought I would have the courage to write a book. I started writing early in my career to decompress and clear my mind of everything I was experiencing at work. Fast-forward eight years and my writing has culminated into what you are holding in your hand. I started the journey, but **WE** made it possible. If you enjoyed this journey we have shared together, please know the credit for its creation has to be shared with so many others. Happiness requires collaboration and words cannot express how grateful I am for all the support, well wishes, social media likes, and messages I have received along the way. If I forget to mention anyone, I apologize—it is not intentional.

First and foremost, I want to thank a very special patient of mine who pushed me to do this; Madeline Niebanck. She was the first person who told me I could and should write a book. If our paths never crossed, I do not think I would have taken this step in sharing the lessons I have learned from my patients with the world. As for the book itself, I want to thank Professor Eric Koester from Georgetown University.

His passion, dedication, and direction during this process instilled a belief in me that I can do this. I also want to acknowledge the team at New Degree Press for the support along the way in making my dream of writing this book a reality. Specifically, Melody Delgado Lorbeer (developmental editor), Amanda Moskowitz (marketing and revisions editor), and Brian Bies (head of publishing).

I would be remiss if I did not acknowledge everyone I interviewed during this process, as well as those who joined me on my Instagram Live segments: Eric LeGrand, Adele Levine, Bonnie Evans, Ashley McKenna, Shannon Motisi, Sean O' Donnell, Jimmy Spiegel, Sydney Welch, Greg Hannah, and Mike Luciano.

I would also like to take a moment and acknowledge my family, friends, and patients who have supported me during my presale campaign. Thank you! Thank you! Thank you! We not only achieved, but exceeded, our goals of raising funds for Team LeGrand in the process:

Judy Fiorilli	Todd Williams
Amanda Hamilton	Cynthia Vlad
John Yoon	Sammy Naffaa
Donna Niebanck	Megan Flynn
Barbara Quinn	Odie Fakhouri
Jennifer Fakhoury	Tiffany Mosher
Matthew Osman	Urmi Basu
Amanda Fakhoury	Suleiman Fakhouri
Dunia Fakhoury	Gabriella Stiefbold
Alexa Rubino	Jillian Rementilla
Semmes Walmsley	Sydney Welch

Nick Del Guercio

Chris and Connie Quinn

Yelena Boltyan

Jessica and AJ Amalfe

Samia and Ole Naffaa

Abigail Reid

Chelsea, James, and Sophie
Pizzillo

Jorge Narvaez

Corey Dunbar

Amal, Samih, and Tamara
Haddad

Christina Yee

David Kietrys

Mike and Laryssa Del Guercio

Leslie Fakhoury

Issa Fakhoury

Laura Mullin

Anthony Cruz

Lorene Hattar

Diala Gammoh

Frank and Kristi Fiorilli

Adam Katzenback

Alexandra Ain

Ed Johnson

Joseph Taylor

Salem El Nimri

Tony Rossi

Gerard Pizzillo

Drew Heinold

Ramez Fakhoury

Mike McCaffery

Herbert Caussade

Laura Heller

Joseph McGinley

Daniel MacDonald

Anthony Haddad

Robbin Cartier

Vera Shekhets and Justin Fox

Stephanie Trstensky

Angie Haddad

Bryan Crandall

Susan and Jerry Pizzillo

Michael Ziarnowski

Justin Pinkerton

Stephanie Yee

Kristin Conway

Hanna Diver

Sami Arida

Conrad Symber

Regina Philipps

Steven and Kristina Indelicato

Carmine Berardi

Lisa Indelicato

Kyle Mullin

Stephen Fredericksen

Eric Koester

Debbie Fakhoury

Heather Monaco

Joe McGinley

Vincent Catellano

Patty and Jim Esposito

Tarek and Haifa Fakhoury

Razan and Geries Tadros

Jakeem Johnson

Jason and Alex Friel

Rebecca Vu

Mona Fakhoury

Christine Cavallo

Shannon Motisi

Daniel Demasters

Olivia Krupinski

Ashley McKenna

Gerard Fluet

Beth Laboranti

Jaime Baynes-Fields

Chad Barbieri

Kregg Laundon

Eileen Rollin

Anthony Giordano

Devon Werner

Bill Whiteside

Ruba Fakhoury

Walid Gammouh

Galina Smirnova

Joseph Donegan

Mike Ferber

Steve Solecki

Laura and Vincent Indelicato

Scott Stansbury

Amanda Sylvester

Luma Fakhoury

Mariuxi Penafiel

Nicole Tahan

Crystal Isaac

Ziyad Fakhoury

Greg and Megan Martinez

Mary Fakhouri

Joseph DeAndrea

Morven Rodrigues

Motaz Alabdalrazzag

Robert Corbin

William Rossy

Prince Adade

Joseph McMahon

Ryan Hayward

Craig and Jessica Langan

Gabriele Gudonaviciute

Diana Gasperoni

Will Ford

Michael Luciano

Debbie Miele

Amir Fakhoury

Juliana Gendelman

Christine Schaub

Dianna Rosario

Dan Durnian

Sean Casey

Laith Qandah

Monica Dasgupta

Michael Cladek

APPENDIX

INTRODUCTION:

Kessler, Henry. *The Knife is Not Enough.* New York: W.W. Norton & Company, 1968.

Frankl, Viktor E. *Man's Search for Meaning.* Boston: Beacon Press, 1959.

Levine, Adele, conversation with author, March 24, 2020.

Ware, Bronnie. *The Top Five Regrets of the Dying: A Life Transformed by the Dearly Departing.* Carlsbad: Hay House, 2012.

CHAPTER 1:

American Physical Therapy Association. "100 Years: 1921-2021—100 Milestones of Physical Therapy: 2000." Accessed June 22, 2020. https://centennial.apta.org/timeline/vision-statement-for-the-physical-therapy-profession-established/.

American Physical Therapy Association. "American Physical Therapy Association History." Accessed June 15, 2020. https://www. apta.org/apta-history.

CHAPTER 2:

Dusek, Jeffery A., Patricia L. Hibberd, Beverly Buczynski, Bei-Hung Chang, KAthryn C. Dusek, Jennifer Johnston, Ann L. Wohlhueter, Herbert Benson, and Randall M. Zusman. "Stress Management versus Lifestyle Modification on Systolic Hypertension and Medication Elimination: A Randomized Trial." *The Journal of Alternative and Complementary Medicine* 14, no. 2 (2008): 129-138. 10.1089/acm.2007.0623.

Rankin, Lisa. "Is There Scientific Proof We Can Heal Ourselves?" December 19, 2012, TED video, 0:45. https://www.youtube. com/watch?v=LWQfe__fNbs&list=PLYSbVjCP2kuite9LX-FeEyz-yp5VYRXKzE.

Santos, Laurie. "You Can Change." September 13, 2019. In *The Happiness Lab.* Produced by Pushkin. Podcast, MP3 audio, 7:30. https://podcasts.apple.com/us/podcast/the-happiness-lab-with-dr-laurie-santos/id1474245040?i=1000449594792.

Santos, Laurie. "Don't Accentuate the Positive." October 29, 2019. In *The Happiness Lab.* Produced by Pushkin. Podcast, MP3 audio, 19:45. https://podcasts.apple.com/us/podcast/the-happiness-lab-with-dr-laurie-santos/id1474245040?i=1000455352101.

Wondrusch, Christine and Corina Schuster-Amft. "A Standardized Motor Imagery Introduction Program (MIIP) for Neuro-rehabilitation: Development and Evaluation." *Frontiers in Human Neuroscience* 7, (August 2013): 477. 10.3389/fnhum.2013.00477.

CHAPTER 3: (PART 1)

Figure 1: Stedanacci, Richard G. "Admission Criteria for Facility-Based Post-Acute Services." *Annals of Long-Term Care: Clinical Care and Aging* 23, no. 11 (2015): 18-20. https://www.managedhealthcareconnect.com/articles/admission-criteria-facility-based-post-acute-services.

Heller, Laura. Email message to author, July 29, 2019.

LeGrand, Eric. Conversation with author, March 27, 2020.

CHAPTER 3: (PART 2)

Amputee Coalition of America. "Limb Loss Statistics," accessed July 15, 2020. https://3w568y1pmc7umeynn206c1my-wpengine.netdna-ssl.com/wp-content/uploads/2020/03/LLAM-Infographic-2020.pdf.

Baub, Jean-Dominique. *The Diving Bell and the Butterfly.* New York: Vintage International, 1997.

Figure 2: National Institute of Health. U.S. National Library of Medicine. "Stroke," accessed April 20, 2020. https://medlineplus.gov/stroke.html.

Figure 3: National Institute of Health. U.S. National Library of Medicine. "Traumatic Brain Injury," accessed June 2, 2020. https://vsearch.nlm.nih.gov/vivisimo/cgi-bin/query-meta?v%3Aproject=medlineplus&v%3Asources=medlineplus-bundle&query=traumatic+brain+injury.

Figure 4: National Institute of Health. U.S. National Library of Medicine. "Limb Loss," accessed July 15, 2020. https://medlineplus.gov/limbloss.html.

Figure 5: National Institute of Health. U.S. National Library of Medicine. "Spinal Cord Injury," accessed June 14, 2020. https://medlineplus.gov/spinalcordinjuries.html.

Motisi, Shannon. Conversation with author, April 15, 2020.

National Institute of Health. U.S. National Library of Medicine. "Traumatic Brain Injury," accessed March 20, 2020. https://vsearch.nlm.nih.gov/vivisimo/cgi-bin/query-meta?v%3Aproject=medlineplus&v%3Asources=medlineplus-bundle&query=traumatic+brain+injury.

Umphred, Darcy. *Neurological Rehabilitation.* St. Louis: Mosby Elsevier, 2007.

CHAPTER 4

Carlson, Ben. "A Wealth of Common Sense." *Perception Matters* (blog), November 13, 2014. https://awealthofcommonsense.com/2014/11/relative/.

Gilbert, D.T. and Timothy D. Wilson. *In Thinking and Feeling: The Role of Affect in Social Cognition.* Cambridge: Cambridge University Press, 2000. https://dash.harvard.edu/bitstream/handle/1/14549983/Miswanting.pdf?sequence=1&isAllowed=y.

Lyubomirsky, Sonja. *The How of Happiness: A New Approach to Getting the Life You Want.* New York: The Penguin Press, 2008.

Santos, Laurie. "The Science of Well-Being." Yale University, 2018. Part One—Rethinking Awesome Stuff, video, 15:00. https://www.coursera.org/learn/the-science-of-well-being/lecture/fnM3M/part-1-rethink-awesome-stuff.

Santos, Laurie. "The Science of Well-Being." Yale University, 2018. Part One—Rethinking Awesome Stuff, video, 1:50. https://www.coursera.org/learn/the-science-of-well-being/lecture/fnM3M/part-1-rethink-awesome-stuff.

Santos, Laurie. "You Can Change," September 13, 2019, in *The Happiness Lab,* produced by Pushkin, podcast, MP3 audio, 21:54. https://podcasts.apple.com/us/podcast/the-happiness-lab-with-dr-laurie-santos/id1474245040?i=1000449594792.

Waldinger, Robert. "What Makes a Good Life? Lessons from the Longest Study on Happiness." November, 2015, TED video, 10:52. https://www.ted.com/talks/robert_waldinger_what_makes_a_good_life_lessons_from_the_longest_study_on_happiness?language=en.

CHAPTER 5:

Candyce H. Kroenke, Laura D. Kubzansky, Eva S. Schernhammer, Michelle D. Holmes, and Ichiro Kawachi. "Social Networks, Social Support, and Survival after Breast Cancer Diagnosis," *Journal of Clinical Oncology* 24, no.7 (March 1, 2006): 1105-1111. https://ascopubs.org/doi/10.1200/JCO.2005.04.2846.

Gladwell, Malcolm. *Outliers: The Story of Success*. New York: Little, Brown, & Company, 2008.

Merriam-Webster s.v. "apathy (*n*.)." Springfield: Merriam Webster, October 7, 2020. https://www.merriam-webster.com/dictionary/apathy.

Merriam-Webster. s.v. "altruism (*n*.)." Springfield: Merriam Webster, October 4, 2020. https://www.merriam-webster.com/dictionary/altruism.

Motisi, Shannon. Conversation with author, April 15, 2020.

O'Donnell, Sean. Conversation with author, March 3, 2020.

Psychology Research and Reference. "Negative-State Relief Model," accessed April 23, 2020. http://psychology.iresearchnet.com/social-psychology/prosocial-behavior/negative-state-relief-model/.

Rankin, Lissa. *Mind Over Medicine: Scientific Proof that You Can Heal Yourself.* Carlsbad: Hay House, Inc., 2013.

Seltzer, Leon. "The Curse of Apathy: Sources and Solutions." *Psychology Today*, April 27, 2016. https://www.psychologytoday.com/us/blog/evolution-the-self/201604/the-curse-apathy-sources-and-solutions.

Seltzer, Leon. "The Curse of Apathy: Sources and Solutions." *Psychology Today*, April 27, 2016. https://www.psychologytoday.com/us/blog/evolution-the-self/201604/the-curse-apathy-sources-and-solutions.

CHAPTER 6:

Duckworth, Angela. *Grit*. New York: Scribner, 2016.

Howes, Lewis. "Embrace Your Struggle with Devon Still." February 27, 2019. In *The School of Greatness*. Podcast, MP3 audio, 44:45. https://podcasts.apple.com/us/podcast/the-school-of-greatness/id596047499?i=1000440881027.

LeGrand, Eric. Conversation with author, March 27, 2020.

Wright, Jay. *Attitude: Develop a Winning Mindset on and off the Court*. New York: Ballentine Books, 2017.

CHAPTER 7:

Evans, Bonnie. Conversation with author, May 12, 2020.

Harvard Health Publishing. Harvard Medical School. "Giving Thanks Can Make You Happier," accessed May 20, 2020. https://www.health.harvard.edu/healthbeat/giving-thanks-can-make-you-happier.

Hospice Foundation of America. "Grief," accessed May 23, 2020. https://web.archive.org/web/20120319211508/http://www.hospicefoundation.org/grief.

Niebanck, Maddie. Conversation with author, March 26, 2020.

Positive Psychology. "The Science and Research on Gratitude and Happiness," accessed May 15, 2020. https://positivepsychology.com/gratitude-happiness-research/.

Steindl-Rast, David. "Want to be Happy? Be Grateful." June 2013, TED video, 5:45. https://www.ted.com/talks/david_steindl_rast_want_to_be_happy_be_grateful?language=en.

Wong Joel Y., Jesse Owen, Nicole T. Gabana, Joshua W. Brown, Sydney McInnis, Paul Toth, and Lynn Gilman. "Does Gratitude Writing Improve the Mental Health of Psychotherapy Clients? Evidence from a randomized controlled trial." *Psychotherapy Research* 28, no. 2 (2016): 192-202. https://www.tandfonline.com/doi/full/10.1080/10503307.2016.1169332?scroll=top&needAccess=true.

Wong Joel Y., Jesse Owen, Nicole T. Gabana, Joshua W. Brown, Sydney McInnis, Paul Toth, and Lynn Gilman. "Does Gratitude Writing Improve the Mental Health of Psychotherapy Clients? Evidence from a randomized controlled trial." *Psychotherapy Research* 28, no. 2 (2016): 192-202. https://www.tandfonline.com/doi/full/10.1080/10503307.2016.1169332?scroll=top&needAccess=true.

Wong Joel Y., Jesse Owen, Nicole T. Gabana, Joshua W. Brown, Sydney McInnis, Paul Toth & Lynn Gilman. "Does Gratitude Writing Improve the Mental Health of Psychotherapy Clients? Evidence from a randomized controlled trial." *Psychotherapy Research* 28, no. 2 (2016): 192-202. https://www.tandfonline.com/doi/full/10.1080/10503307.2016.1169332?scroll=top&needAccess=true.

CHAPTER 8:

Clear, James. *Atomic Habits*. New York: Penguin Random House, 2018.

Coelho, Paulo. *The Pilgrimage.* San Francisco: Harper One, 2008.

Goodreads. "Quotable Quote," accessed October 2, 2020. https://www.goodreads.com/quotes/222770-true-happiness-is-to-enjoy-the-present-without-anxious-dependence.

Johnson, Inky (@inkyjohnson), Instagram photo, August 17, 2020. https://www.instagram.com/p/CEAJFMwsFh6/.

Mylett, Ed. "Perspective Drives Performance with Inky Johnson." February 5, 2020. In *The Ed Mylett Show.* Podcast, MP3 audio, 33:30. https://luminarypodcasts.com/listen/ed-mylett-047/ed-mylett-show/perspective-drives-performance-w-inky-johnson/698d38ce-7894-4d54-a737-0b18ae327e82?country=US.

Niebanck, Maddie. Conversation with author, March 26, 2020.

Taylor, Jill Bolte. *My Stroke of Insight.* New York: The Penguin Group, 2006.

Van Schneider, Tobias. "If You Want It, You Might Get It. The Reticular Activating System Explained." *Desk of Van Schneider* (blog), June 22, 2017. https://medium.com/desk-of-van-schneider/if-you-want-it-you-might-get-it-the-reticular-activating-system-explained-761b6ac14e53.

CHAPTER 9:

Cedars-Sinai. "The Science of Kindness," accessed April 17, 2020. https://www.cedars-sinai.org/blog/science-of-kindness.html.

Mylett, Ed. "Perspective Drives Performance with Inky Johnson." February 5, 2020. In *The Ed Mylett Show*. Podcast, MP3 audio, 27.00. https://luminarypodcasts.com/listen/ed-mylett-047/ed-mylett-show/perspective-drives-performance-w-inky-johnson/698d38ce-7894-4d54-a737-0b18ae327e82?country=US.

Niebanck, Maddie. Conversation with author, March 26, 2020.

Newton, Alan. "Practicing Intoku." *Executive Secretary Magazine*, November 25, 2017. https://executivesecretary.com/practising-intoku/#:~:text=Intoku%20is%20a%20Japanese%20word,secretly%2C%20for%20its%20own%20sake.

CHAPTER 10:

Howes, Lewis. "Building Human Connection in a Digital World." November 11, 2018. In *The School of Greatness*. Podcast, video, 7:40. https://www.youtube.com/watch?v=S6zjkKL93PQ.

Howes, Lewis. "Building Human Connection in a Digital World." November 11, 2018. In *The School of Greatness*. Podcast, video, 5:20. https://www.youtube.com/watch?v=S6zjkKL93PQ.

Howes, Lewis. "The Art of Human Connection." October 29, 2019. In *The School of Greatness*. Podcast, video, 24:25. https://www.youtube.com/watch?v=iCi1WuyAhhw.

Howes, Lewis. "The Art of Human Connection." October 29, 2019. In *The School of Greatness*. Podcast, video, 24:50. https://www.youtube.com/watch?v=iCi1WuyAhhw.

Queen Rania. "Queen Rania Speaks with Oprah on Oprah Show." May 17, 2006. Video, 1:20. https://www.youtube.com/watch?v=iIKI8WX8Btw.

Santos, Laurie. "Mistakenly Seeking Solitude." October 8, 2019. In *The Happiness Lab*, produced by Pushkin. Podcast, MP3 audio, 7:30. https://podcasts.apple.com/us/podcast/the-happiness-lab-with-dr-laurie-santos/id1474245040?i=1000452731206.

Schawbel, Dan (@danschawbel), Instagram photo, January 21, 2020. https://www.instagram.com/p/B7tVahtpFHH/.

Voice Message to author. November 30, 2018.

CHAPTER 11:

LeGrand, Eric. Conversation with author, March 27, 2020.

Merriam-Webster. s.v. "normal (*adj.*)." Springfield: Merriam Webster, September 29, 2020, https://www.merriam-webster.com/dictionary/normal?src=search-dict-hed.

St. John, Bonnie. Lecture October 11, 2018 at Seton Hall University. https://www.shu.edu/news/paralympic-medalist-bonnie-st-john-on-campus-oct-11.cfm.

Santos, Laurie. "The Science of Well-Being." Yale University, 2018. Part One—Thwart hedonic Adaptation, video, 1:50. https://www.coursera.org/learn/the-science-of-well-being/lecture/EVVHW/part-2-thwart-hedonic-adaptation.

CHAPTER 12:

Irvine, William B. *The Stoic Challenge: A Philosophers Guide to Becoming Tougher, Calmer, and More Resilient.* New York: W. W. Norton & Company, Inc, 2019.

Merriam-Webster, s.v. "dead (*adj.*)." Springfield: Merriam Webster, October 6, 2020, https://www.merriam-webster.com/dictionary/dead.

Waldinger, Robert. "What Makes a Good Life? Lessons from the Longest Study on Happiness." November, 2015, TED video, 8:54. https://www.ted.com/talks/robert_waldinger_what_makes_a_good_life_lessons_from_the_longest_study_on_happiness?language=en.

Made in the USA
Middletown, DE
20 May 2021